# The Skeptical Professional's Guide to Rational Prescribing

# The Skeptical Professional's Guide to Rational Prescribing

## The Impact of Scientific Fraud and Misconduct

### Charles E. Dean, MD

Staff without Compensation
Minneapolis Veterans Administration Medical Center
Minneapolis, Minnesota

Voting Member
Institutional Review Board
Pharmacy and Therapeutics Committee

Author of *The Skeptical Professional's Guide to Psychiatry:
On the Risks and Benefits of Antipsychotics, Antidepressants,
Psychiatric Diagnoses, and Neuromania* (Routledge, 2021)

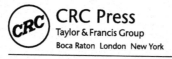

**CRC Press**
Taylor & Francis Group
Boca Raton  London  New York

CRC Press is an imprint of the
Taylor & Francis Group, an **informa** business

First edition published 2022
by CRC Press
6000 Broken Sound Parkway NW, Suite 300, Boca Raton, FL 33487-2742

and by CRC Press
4 Park Square, Milton Park, Abingdon, Oxon, OX14 4RN

*CRC Press is an imprint of Taylor & Francis Group, LLC*

---

**Library of Congress Cataloging-in-Publication Data**

Names: Dean, Charles E., author.
Title: The skeptical professional's guide to rational prescribing : the impact of scientific fraud and misconduct / by Charles E. Dean.
Description: First edition. | Boca Raton, FL : CRC Press, 2022. | Includes bibliographical references and index. | Summary: "The raging COVID-19 pandemic has shaken our trust in science. Contents are set in a clinical context, wherein misconduct and fraud affect rational prescribing, a process that depends on balancing the risk-benefit ratio of treatments, whether pharmacologic or psychotherapeutic"–Provided by publisher.
Identifiers: LCCN 2021062205 (print) | LCCN 2021062206 (ebook) | ISBN 9781032211930 (hbk) | ISBN 9781032211923 (pbk) | ISBN 9781003267218 (ebk)
Subjects: MESH: Inappropriate Prescribing | Drug Prescriptions | Scientific Misconduct | Pharmaceutical Research | United States
Classification: LCC RS57 (print) | LCC RS57 (ebook) | NLM QV 748 | DDC 615.1/4–dc23/eng/20220113
LC record available at https://lccn.loc.gov/2021062205
LC ebook record available at https://lccn.loc.gov/2021062206

---

ISBN: 978-1-032-21193-0 (hbk)
ISBN: 978-1-032-21192-3 (pbk)
ISBN: 978-1-003-26721-8 (ebk)

DOI: 10.1201/9781003267218

Typeset in Minion
by KnowledgeWorks Global Ltd.

# Dedication

*To Horace Freeland Judson, Elliot Valenstein, Robert Whitaker, Carl Elliott, and Marcia Angell whose work on fraud, misconduct, and ethics has been an inspiration.*

The author will donate any royalties to the Fisher House at the Minneapolis VA Medical Center.

# Contents

# Author

**Dr. Dean** has his residency training in psychiatry at the University of Cincinnati. He then volunteered for service in the US Army Medical Corp and was stationed at the 2nd General Hospital in Landstuhl, West Germany from 1965 to 1968, followed by 13 years at the Hennepin County Medical Center in Minneapolis, Minnesota. He had a short stint in private practice, then joined the Minneapolis VA Medical Center in 1987. In 2012, he retired from clinical practice but has remained a voting member of the Institutional Review Board and the Pharmacy and Formulary Committee. He has won seven Teacher of the Year awards from the Department of Psychiatry at the University of Minnesota, where he developed and taught courses in clinical neuroscience and psychopharmacology. His primary research interests have been in tardive dyskinesia, diagnoses, psychotropic medications, and the history of psychiatry. Recent publications include "Neural Circuitry and Precision Medicines for Mental Disorders: Are They Compatible? "Whither Research Domain Criteria?" "Personality Disorders as a Basis for Discharge and Denial of Benefits in the Military. Logical or Abusive?" His first book was *The Skeptical Professional's Guide to Psychiatry: On the Risks and Benefits of Antipsychotics, Antidepressants, Psychiatric Diagnoses, and Neuromania*, published in 2021.

# List of Abbreviations

| | |
|---|---|
| **APA** | American Psychiatric Association |
| **BMC** | BioMed Central |
| **CONSORT** | Consolidated Standards of Reporting Trials |
| **COIs** | Conflicts of interest |
| **COPE** | Committee on Publication Ethics |
| **DCTA** | Direct-to Consumer Advertising |
| **DSM** | *Diagnostic and Statistical Manual*, APA |
| **DOAJ** | Directory of Open Access Journals |
| **EBM** | Evidence-based medicine |
| **ENIGMA** | Enhancing neuroimaging genetics through meta-analysis |
| **EQUATOR** | Enhancing the quality and transparency of research |
| **FCOIs** | Financial conflicts of interest |
| **FDA** | Food and Drug Administration |
| **ICMJE** | International Committee of Medical Journal Editors |
| **JAMA** | *Journal of the American Medical Association* |
| **NIH** | National Institutes of Health |
| **NIMH** | National Institute of Mental Health |
| **OI** | Open innovation |
| **ORI** | Office of Research Integrity |
| **OSI** | Office of Scientific Integrity |
| **PRISMA** | Preferred reporting items for systematic reviews and meta-analyses |
| **PTIE** | Promotion and Tenure-Innovation and Entrepreneurialship Coalition |
| **PRO** | Reporting patient outcomes |
| **RCTs** | Randomized controlled trials |
| **TOP** | Transparency and Openness Promotion Guideline |
| **UIC** | University-industry collaboration |

# Introduction: Historical Roots and Recurrence

## Introduction

In 2020, clinicians, patients, and families find themselves in the middle of a battle featuring on the one hand a growing number of citizens who distrust science, and, on the other, those who maintain that science is our primary hope for survival, not only with regard to the COVID-19 pandemic, but climate change. This battle is taking place in the context of a deeply polarized society, with markedly different perceptions regarding the adequacy of the health care system, the risks vs benefits of vaccines, and whether masking and social distancing are acceptable steps in ameliorating the pandemic, despite significant evidence documenting their positive effects. Another divisive issue: the role of racism in our failure to achieve comparable outcomes across the population.

At the same time, science itself is in the middle of a struggle over the causes and consequences of scientific misconduct and outright fraud. The struggle is not new, as documented in Broad and Wade's 1982 volume, *Betrayers of the Truth: Fraud and Deceit in the Halls of Science*,[1] where they documented cases of fraud beginning in the 2nd century BC. A number of these involved eminences such as Galileo, Mendel, and Admiral Peary. Not surprisingly, several of the accusations involving Ptolemy, Hipparchus, Newton, and Robert Millikan were refuted in 1991 by a physicist at the California Institute of Technology.[2] Nevertheless, in 2004, H.F. Judson added more examples in his book, *The Great Betrayal: Fraud in Science*,[3] where he described an extensive culture of fraud in science, business, and other fields. As we shall see, a number of steps have been taken to correct scientific misconduct, but during the past decade we have seen many instances of flagrant misconduct and research fraud, a number of which have taken place in our most prominent universities and hospitals.

In one instance, Dr. Piera Anversa, a well-known cardiovascular investigator, at Harvard and Brigham and Women's Hospital, claimed in 2000 that he could regenerate damaged cardiac tissue by injecting bone-marrow derived stem cells into the hearts of mice, with the stem cells turning into cardiac cells.[4,5] Since death from cardiac disease is the number one cause of death in the United States,[6] his research led to the formation of several start-up companies, and an NIH-funded clinical trial. However, efforts at duplicating his work failed. Despite growing doubts in the scientific community, he proceeded to publish some 31 articles, claiming that critics simply did not understand how to duplicate his work. In 2013, Harvard and Brigham and Women's Hospital began to investigate. Four years later, Brigham paid the government $10 million to settle claims that Dr. Anvsersa and his lab had fraudulently obtained research funding from the National Institutes of Health (NIH).[4] In 2018, Harvard and Brigham noted that the 31 articles should be retracted.[5] Nevertheless, a clinical trial funded by the National

DOI: 10.1201/9781003267218-1

Heart, Lung, and Blood Institute began injecting stem cells into patients with heart failure, despite research showing that injected stem cells remained stem cells.[4]

In 2019, the *New York Times*[7] reported that Duke University agreed to pay the federal government $112.5 million to settle claims that investigators had submitted falsified data in its efforts to win more than two dozen grants from the NIH and the Environmental Protection Agency. It appears that the falsified data was not discovered by the granting agencies and their reviewers. Instead, a whistle-blower at Duke had filed a lawsuit claiming that an investigator had submitted fabricated data in the course of receiving $200 million in federal grants. The investigator was fired in 2018 for embezzling funds and submitting forged documents. Duke then announced in 2019 that it will create an advisory panel on research integrity.[7]

In another case, an investigation by the *New York Times* and *ProPublica*[8] revealed that the chief medical officer at Memorial Sloan Kettering Cancer Institute, Dr. José Baselga, had failed to follow financial disclosure rules posted by the American Association for Cancer Research when he was president of the organization. He also failed to acknowledge payments from companies associated with cancer research in his many papers published by the journal, *Cancer Discovery*—although he was one of the two editors! In addition, he was accused of spinning the results of two trials sponsored by Roche, a company that had paid him at least $3 million in consulting fees from 2014 and subsequently. Dr. Baselga also served on the boards of at least six companies, thus incurring a fiduciary responsibility to advance the interests of those companies. During the years 2013 to 2017, he took in almost $3.5 million from nine companies. In a review of his publications, the *Times* and *ProPublica* found that he had not mentioned his industry relationships in 60%. In 2017, he failed to acknowledge his ties to industry in 87% of the papers he had authored or co-authored. He promised to correct these omissions in 17 of the publications. Why not the rest?

A spokesperson for Sloan Kettering stated that Dr. Baselga had informed the center of his relationships with industry, but that it was his responsibility to submit such information to the journals.[8] Despite this rather cavalier attitude, Sloan Kettering announced in 2019 that it was restricting its top executives from serving on the boards of drug companies,[9] and that its CEO had resigned from the board of Merck—which had paid him $300,000 in 2017! In addition, Sloan Kettering ruled that its employees cannot accept equity stocks or other forms of personal compensation from companies. We should note too that Dr. Baselga had resigned from Sloan Kettering shortly after the *New York Times* article appeared, but was quickly hired by another drug company. In December of 2020, the *New York Times* reported[10] that Sloan Kettering had paid Dr. Baselga more than $1.5 million in severance pay in 2018 and 2019. Despite this history, he is now an executive at AstraZeneca, where he oversees the development of drugs aimed at treating cancer.

Then we have the story of Professor Sid Gilman, a former chair of the Neurology Department at the University of Michigan, who in 2012 was accused by the Securities Exchange Commission (SEC) of participating in an insider trading scheme.[11] Dr. Gilman had become involved in an "expert network firm," Gerson Lehman, an arrangement whereby medical experts in various fields are hired to supply information to hedge funds and other entities. In this case, Dr. Gilman was paid some $100,000 to pass on information to a hedge fund manager about a clinical trial of a new drug for Alzheimer's disease. When the trial failed, he kept up his end of the bargain by relaying the results to the portfolio manager. The firm proceeded to sell the company's stock and thereby avoid almost $300 million in losses. Dr. Gilman resigned from the University of Michigan, but signed a non-prosecution agreement with the SEC after agreeing to testify. He paid $234,000 to settle the lawsuit.[11]

In a related report, Timmerman and Heath, reporters at the *Seattle Times*,[12] noted that the Gerson Lehman group had signed 60,000 physicians who had agreed with work with Wall Street. During their investigation into the MD-Wall Street connections, the reporters found 26 cases in which physicians leaked confidential—and sometimes critical information—regarding their drug trials to investment firms. The reporters interviewed 15 of the participants in these schemes, who denied any wrongdoing, despite charging $300–$500 hourly to speak with investors.

Arthur Caplan, a bioethicist, who was asked to comment on the practice,[12] said it is a moral cesspool, and the last straw in the corporatization of American medicine. Well, it was not the last straw. Indeed, the COVID-19 pandemic has led to additional instances of misconduct. While the pandemic has resulted in hundreds of papers on SARS-CoV-2, including its molecular structure, longer-term effects, risk factors, and fatalities, it has also led to considerable pressure on the scientific community to come up with recommendations for treatment and the rapid development of vaccines. Indeed, the potential rewards, both financial and academic, are immense. Unfortunately, two highly publicized papers, one published by the *New England Journal of Medicine* (*NEJM*),[13] and the other by the *Lancet*,[14] (cited here in its retracted version) came under severe criticism by hundreds of scientists worldwide.

The article in the *NEJM* by MR Mehra et al.[13] focused on cardiovascular disease, drug therapy, and mortality in hospitalized patients with a confirmed diagnosis of COVID-19. The numbers were huge: 8,819 patients from 169 hospitals in Asia, North America, and Europe that were participating in an international registry using electronic patient data. The authors noted that underlying cardiovascular disease was associated with an increased risk of death, but did not find an association between in-hospital deaths and treatment with angiotensin-converting enzyme-2 inhibitors, or angiotensin receptor inhibitors.

These were important results, given conflicting recommendations about the use of these drugs in COVID-19. However, a highly critical open letter[15] soon appeared, and was addressed to the study authors and Eric Ruben, the editor-in-chief of the *NEJM*. It was signed by some 174 scientists from Africa, Asia, Europe, and North America. This "Expression of concern regarding data integrity and results" noted difficulties in reconciling the UK and Turkey data obtained from the Surgisphere Corporation with publicly available government data. In addition, the estimated age-dependent mortality did *not* show the expected increase in patients over 60, inconsistent with other data. The signatories recommended an independent validation of the data from the Surgisphere database, and sought assurances that the data had been collected legally and ethically. Dr. Rubin replied, stating that he has asked the authors show evidence that the data are reliable.[16]

Many of the same concerns were raised with regard to a study in the *Lancet*[14,17] examining the use of hydrochloroquine or chloroquine with or without a macrolide for treatment of COVID-19. The authors, three of whom were investigators on the *NEJM* study, used the same Surgisphere database. Again, the numbers were huge: 96,032 hospitalized COVID-19 patients from six continents. Their data showed a 30% increase in the risk of excessive deaths and ventricular arrhythmias associated with the use each drug regimen, a potentially important finding.

However, this study also prompted an open letter[18] to the authors and Richard Horton, editor of the *Lancet*, where the several hundred signatories cast doubt on the statistical analyses, the lack of an ethics review, the use of data incompatible with government reports, and "unusually small reported variation in baseline variables, interventions and outcomes between continents." The critics asked Professor Mehra for the raw data, but he refused, saying the data sharing agreements with governments, countries, and hospitals do not allow data sharing. The signatories also called for independent validation of the data, additional statistical analyses, and publication of the comments from peer reviewers who recommended publication. Others[18] have pointed out that the lead co-author of the *Lancet* study, Sapan Desai, is the founder and CEO of the Surgisphere corporation, has refused to identify the participating hospitals and the countries. Dr. Mehra, the lead author of both the *Lancet* and the *NEJM* studies, is a director at Brigham and Women's Hospital, which funded the *Lancet* study. (For more on COVID-19, see Chapter 9.)

The conflicts of interest in these studies are obvious, as is the lack of transparency, yet the peer reviewers and the editors of the *Lancet* and the *NEJM* somehow overlooked these problems, and allowed publication. (These papers have continued to be cited, despite being retracted, with 52% of recent citations failing to mention the retractions.[19]) Why and how did that happen? Part of the answer appears to be the sheer size of the studies, and the alleged diversity of the populations, not to speak of the aforementioned pressure to come up with some definitive answers regarding treatment, hospitalizations, and mortality. Did the peer reviewers cast any doubt on the validity of the studies? Did they make any suggestions regarding the content and statistical analyses? Did the editors have any doubts about the validity of the studies? Were there dissenting voices on the editorial boards? If so, how was this handled? (I will have much more to say about the peer-review process in a later chapter.)

Although we have largely focused on fraud and misconduct in the United States, other countries have had similar problems. For example, a new study by the Dutch National Survey[20] on Research Integrity attempted to survey over 60,000 Dutch scientists with regard to fraud and less serious but still questionable research practices, but only 6800 returned the survey, apparently fearing negative publicity. Still, this is the largest survey on record. Sadly, 8% reported fabrication or falsification of research results, about double the rate found in previous studies. With regard to other less serious but questionable practices, 53% of PhD students admitted such behavior, as did 49% of associate and full professors.

One of the more disturbing findings from this introductory review is the frequency with which reports of fraud originated from whistle-blowers, outside investigators, and journalists. How did the funding agencies, such as the NIH, with their draconian peer-review processes led by international experts, fail to discover the fraudulent data contained in the two dozen grants obtained by Duke? Why did the Sloan Kettering Institute allow its chief medical officer to continue in his advisory role to multiple drug companies, and deny any conflicts of interest across multiple studies? Did no one at Sloan Kettering read his papers? That seems unlikely, so we are left with the conclusion that his behavior was tolerated due to the massive amounts of money and fame that he brought to the institution.

These reports contain the essence of the issues confronting science today, including untoward ties with drug companies, the power of the pharmaceutical industry to co-opt physicians and institutions, the failure of peer review, the use of fraudulent data, and the failure of institutions to monitor their investigators. However, other topics are also in need of review, including publication bias, spinning poor or questionable results into positive outcomes, omitting or changing he primary outcomes of studies after the data fail to deliver the expected results, the use of ghost and guest authors, and excessive reliance on meta-analyses, which, as we shall see, have their own biases.

Unfortunately, scientific misconduct and fraud are major barriers to clinicians who seek to balance the risk–benefit ratio for their treatment recommendations. This step is especially critical in psychiatry, given the lack of any objective, clinically useful biomarkers helpful in establishing the validity of a mental disorder.[21,22] Remarkably, Lewis Judd, the former director of the National Institute of Mental Health (NIMH), claimed in a 1990 interview[23] that psychiatrists can diagnose mental disorders with the same certainty that other doctors can diagnose diabetes or arthritis. Nonsense. He seemed to forget that internists and other specialists have multiple laboratory and x-ray studies that are available for the validation of each diagnosis. In 2020, psychiatry has none, so we still depend on a synthesis of the history, observations, and the scientific literature in formulating a treatment approach. If the literature is contaminated by misconduct and fraud, the validity of the risk–benefit ratio is compromised. I intend to review these various forms of fraud, their impact on the risk–benefit ratio, and offer recommendations on how recognize misconduct and fraud. While these steps may help, the major problems lie in our profit-driven health care system and the drive for power, money, and fame.

# References

1. Broad, W, et al. *Betrayers of the Truth: Fraud and Deceit in the Halls of Science.* Simon & Schuster, New York, 1982.
2. Goodstein, D. Scientific fraud. *American Scholar.* Autumn 1991.
3. Judson, HF. *The Great Betrayal. Fraud in Science.* Harcourt, Inc., Orlando, 2004.
4. Kolata, G. Cardiologist falsified data, Harvard says. *New York Times,* National Edition, October 16, 2018.
5. Kolata, G. His promise to heal bad hearts relied on mountain of false data. *New York Times,* National Edition, October 30, 2018.
6. Dieleman, JL, et al. U.S. spending on personal health care and public bad hearts relied on mountain of false data. *JAMA* 2016.
7. Kaplan, S. Duke to pay $112.5 million over claim it falsified data. *New York Times,* National Edition, March 26, 2019.
8. Ornstein, C, et al. A top doctor didn't disclose corporate ties. *New York Times,* National Edition, September 9, 2018.
9. Thomas, K, et al. Shaken by scandals, cancer institution restricts ties to industry. *New York Times,* National Edition, January 12, 2019.
10. Thomas, K, et al. Sloan Kettering paid $1.5 million to doctor who was forced out over conflicts. *New York Times,* National Edition, December 23, 2020.
11. Rubenfire, AA, et al. Embroiled in scandal, neurology professor retires. *Michigan Daily,* November 28, 2012.
12. Timmerman, L, et al. Drug researchers leak secrets to Wall Street. https://special.seattletimes.com/o/html/businesstechnology/drugsecrets1.html
13. Mehra, MR, et al. Cardiovascular disease, drug therapy, and mortality in COVID-19. *New England Journal of Medicine* 2020. https://doi.org/10.1056/NEJMoa2007621
14. Mehra, MR, et al. Retracted. Hydroxychloroquine or chloroquine with or without a macrolide for treatment of COVID-19: a multinational registry analysis. *Lancet* 2020. https://doi.org/10.1016/S0140-6736(20)31180-6
15. Watson, JA, et al. On behalf of 174 signatories (2020, June 2). An open letter to Mehra, et al. and the *New England Journal of Medicine* (version 1). *Zenodo.* http://doi.org/10.5281/zenodo.3873178
16. Rubin, EJ. Expression of concern: Mehra et al. Cardiovascular disease, drug therapy, and mortality in Covid-19. *New England Journal of Medicine.* http://doi.org/10.1056/NEJMoa200762. June 18, 2020. Doi: 10.1056/NEJMoa2007621
17. Funck-Brentano, et al. Retracted: chloroquine or hydroxychloroquine for COVID-19: why might they be hazardous? *Lancet* 2020. https://doi.org/10.1016/S0140-6736(20)31174-0
18. Watson, J, et al. An open letter to Mehra et al. and the *Lancet* (version 4). 2020. *Zenodo.* http://doi.org/10.5281/zenodo.3871094
19. Piller, C. Disgraced COVID-19 studies are still routinely cited. *Science* 2021.

20. de Vrieze, J. Large survey finds questionable research practices are common. Dutch study finds 8% of scientists have committed fraud. *Science* 2021. Additional details can be found in Gopalakrishna G, et al. Prevalence of questionable research practices, research misconduct, and their potential explanatory factors: a survey among academic researchers in the Netherlands. http://osf.io/vk9yt/

21. First, MB. Paradigm shifts and the development of the *Diagnostic and Statistical Manual of Mental Disorders:* past experiences and future aspirations. *Canadian Journal of Psychiatry* 2010.

22. Zachar, P, et al. The aspirations for a paradigm shift in DSM-5: an oral history. *Journal of Nervous and Mental Disease* 2019.

23. Beecher, LH. A national director of sound mind. Lee H. Beecher, M.D., interviews Lewis L. Judd, M.D., for *Minnesota Medicine* 1990.

# Regulations, the Growth of Pharma, and Diagnostic Expansion, 1951–2013
## *A Wealth Trifecta*

## Introduction

In order to understand the context in which institutions and investigators have been enmeshed in a culture of misconduct, we must examine the development of the medical-industrial complex, a phenomenon that developed very slowly during the 18th and 19th centuries, but then accelerated in the 1950s. The early history of this transition has been described in detail by Paul Starr.[1] In the 18th century, physicians were held in little regard and had no organizational power. During the early 19th century, medicine in general lacked any significant claim to trust on the part of the public, leading families to provide much of the care for those who became ill. However, by the middle of the 19th century, science had provided evidence for the bacterial origin of tuberculosis, cholera, typhoid, and other infectious diseases, eventually leading to laboratory tests that could identify the organisms. In 1905, the spirochete responsible for syphilis was identified, while the Wasserman test for syphilis was introduced in 1906.[1, p.137] This was a very significant development, given the number of cases in the asylums, and a significant boost for the reputation of physicians and their role as caregivers. However, the early psychiatrists, often labeled "alienists," did not fare so well, given their isolation in the burgeoning system of asylums, and the often toxic and brutal therapies inflicted on the patients, including surgical removal of the uterus, teeth, and sections of the gut, extreme waterboarding, injections of horse serum and malarial parasites, cold showers, hyperthermia, restraints, and physical abuse.[2,3]

Nevertheless, advances in science spurred a transition in medical care from the household to the market, or, as Starr put it, the conversion of health care into a commodity, a conversion that led to specialization of labor, more distancing between the ill and their caregivers, and a shift in the number of caregivers to men.[1, p.22] By the mid-20th century, 26% of physicians were employed by institutions. Given the demands on their time and expertise, they began to develop more interest in research and teaching. At the same time, and somewhat paradoxically, physicians moved to enhance their status and financial interests by an anti-organizational stance. As the years passed, physicians railed against health insurance, health-maintenance organizations, and other forms of organized medicine but became enamored with the wealth of the pharmaceutical companies.

Indeed, a vast research structure had begun to develop as early as the 1930s, with the founding of the National Institutes of Health in 1930 and the National Cancer Institute in 1937.[1, p.340]

DOI: 10.1201/9781003267218-2

We must recognize as well the rise of the drug companies that occurred prior to the landmark regulations we will review shortly. From the 1940s to the 1950s, the 15 largest drug companies had 80% of the sales and 90% of the profits.[4] In 1945, Pharma began to increase its investment in research, spending some $40 million, vs $25 million from foundations, universities, and other sources.[1, p.339] By 1959, investment in research and development by Pharma reached $170 million,[5, pp.68–69] but sales, profits, and investment in research would increase dramatically over the next several decades.

## Regulations and legislative landmarks

In 1951, the U.S. Food and Drug Administration (FDA) decreed that new medications were to be available by prescription only.[6] This was a seismic change from the previous centuries that were awash in homemade cures and potions available to anyone. No prescription was needed, despite the toxic ingredients, including mercury, cocaine, opium, and lithium. As Gerald Posner has noted,[7, pp.6–9] these compounds, some 50,000 of them, were often labeled as "miracle cures," with sales eventually reaching $100 million yearly.[7, p.24] In addition, the many small manufacturers of these compounds competed with the burgeoning pharmaceutical industry of the 19th century, which included Squibb, Wyeth, Eli Lilly, and Burroughs Wellcome. These companies heavily invested in developing and promoting opiate-based pain remedies, and, in the case of Merck, promoting cocaine for a variety of ailments, including depression, asthma, and dental pain. At one point, cocaine was listed in the top five best-selling drugs. Similarly, in 2020, we find a resurgence of interest in opioids for treatment-resistant depression and psychedelics (psilocybin, mescaline, ketamine, 3,4 methylenedioxyamphetamine [MDMA] for an ever-expanding list of psychiatric disorders).[8]

The 1951 requirement by the FDA resulted in the transfer of additional power to physicians and Pharma, and the rapid development of psychotropic drugs. These included meprobamate (Equanil) in 1955, followed shortly by antipsychotics, antidepressants, and additional anxiolytics, notably chlordiazepoxide (Librium) in 1960 and diazepam (Valium) in 1963.[2] During the 1960s, chlordiazepoxide was the best-selling drug in the United States, a marker of the upward trend in industry wealth. In 1962, amendments to the Food, Drug, and Cosmetic Act mandated that new drugs were to be aimed at specific disease states, further stimulating growth of the medical-industrial complex, and the transition to a biologically oriented psychiatry.[2] The specificity of disease, however, was not a new idea. Indeed, Thomas Syndenham in the 17th century had advocated that we consider illnesses as specific entities.[9] As I have shown, the search for the specificity of disease and treatment, based on the classic medical model, forced psychiatry into a position where it had to show progress in the area, despite the obstacles,[10,11] meaning more dependence on Pharma and its wealth.

The passage of the Bayh-Dole Act in 1980 was another benchmark, in that it gave universities and biotechnology companies the power to patent discoveries,[12] even if the research had been sponsored by the National Institutes of Health (NIH), which at that time was the primary provider of tax dollars for research. As Marcia Angell, the former editor of the *New England Journal of Medicine* (*NEJM*), has noted,[12] Bayh-Dole was a bonanza for Pharma, and fertilized the growing collaboration between academia and Pharma. Indeed, the editor of *NEJM* expressed his concern in 2004 over the advent of the medical-industrial complex,[13] but this was 20 years after Bayh-Dole, far too late.

Yet another boost for Pharma and prescribers was the appearance of the 3rd edition of the *Diagnostic and Statistical Manual of the American Psychiatric Association,* the DSM-III,[14] an enterprise that expanded the number of diagnosable mental disorders to 265. Only 7 years earlier, the Feighner research criteria[15] had stressed that the scientific literature permitted the diagnosis of only 16 disorders, while the DSM-I of 1952,[16] had specified 106. The DSM-III acknowledged that most disorders had no valid information on their course, treatment, or pathophysiology. Despite misgivings over the epidemic of mental disorders,[17,18] subsequent editions continued to expand the numbers of diagnoses, reaching some 350 in the DSM-5 of 2013.[19]

While the DSM-III was the subject of multiple critiques[20,21] regarding its consensus-based approach and the use of diagnostic checklists (operationalized criteria), the advent of 265 sanctioned diagnoses gave psychiatrists an unprecedented opportunity to increase their prescriptions for psychotropic drugs. As a corollary, DSM-III also provided Pharma an opportunity to increase its neurobiological research into a host of relatively new disorders—fertile ground indeed, since most had no valid information on their course, treatment, or pathophysiology.[14] Nor was there any evidence of an objective, independent biomarker that could validate a diagnosis, a statement true in 2021, despite 60 years of increasingly complex neurobiological research.[22,23]

In 1984, Congress provided Pharma with another bonanza by passing the Drug Competition and Patent Restoration Act (Hatch-Waxman) that added another 5 years of patent protection,[12] and even more time if regulatory delay had stymied marketing. This resulted in another 20 years of patent protection for new drugs, a huge boost for profits. As Mike Magee has noted in his new book, *Code Blue*,[5, p.195] this level of protection was a trade-off involving generic drug manufacturers, who were now allowed to bypass biological testing of generics and simply demonstrate biologic equivalency. But this was not the end of patent protection tactics, with the FDA Modernization Act of 1997 adding another 6 months of protection if the drug had been tested in children.[12]

Whatever the advantages for consumers with regard to generics, the FDA in 1997 proceeded to loosen the restrictions on direct-to-consumer advertising (DTCA), quickly leading to a 300% increase in funds from Pharma aimed at DTCA. By 2002, the profit margins for the ten American drug companies listed in the Fortune 500 were far higher than in any other industry.[12,13] From 2004 to 2011, Pharma began to shift its funding away from basic research, and toward Phase III clinical trials, resulting in a 36% increase by 2011,[24] a shift which continued to increase Pharma's entanglement with academic investigators. Indeed, the share of research funding from the industry grew from 46% in 1994 to 58% in 2012. In the meantime, the NIH aimed the majority of its funding toward basic research.[24]

## Money without limits

In 2015, an analysis[25] of revenue, wholesale pricing, and prescription volume for the 30 top-selling drugs sold in U.S. pharmacies in 2010–2014 found that revenue rose by 61%, reaching $67.3 billion. However, the number of prescriptions rose by only 20%, indicating that the 76% increase in prices was the key factor in boosting revenue. Overall, spending on personal health care (hospital care, clinical services, retail pharmacy sales) reached $2.9 trillion in 2014, a very substantial increase compared with such spending in 1996.[26] In 2014, people in the United States filled at least 4 billion prescriptions, but that number did not include the use of some 300,000 legal, over-the-counter drugs. Those costs are difficult to determine but are estimated at $4 billion yearly.[27, pp.20-33]

In the aggregate, $30.1 trillion was spent on personal health care, 1996–2013.[27] Pharma and psychiatry certainly did well in 2013, with personal health care spending on depressive disorders reaching $71 billion, ranking 6th among 155 medical conditions. Indeed, this surpassed spending on anxiety disorders ($29 billion), attention deficit hyperactivity disorder (ADHD; $23 billion), and schizophrenia ($17.6 billion). Yet, Pharma is working hard to grow its wealth, spending some $280 million on Capitol Hill in 2017, with 1,100 federal lobbyists prowling the halls of Congress.[5, p.22] The FDA continued to help, adding over 20 new indications for antidepressants between 2005 and 2013,[28] while expansion of Medicaid under the Affordable Care Act, and the rapid development of Pharmacy Benefit Managers added both costs and opportunities for patients, physicians, and Pharma.[5]

In the meantime, Pharma continues to claim the cost of research and development that justifies both the high cost of drugs in the United States and the money spent on advertising.[29] However, research at the Institute for Health and Socio-Economic Policy found that of the top 100 drug companies by sales in 2015, 64 companies spent twice as much on marketing and sales as they did on research and development, while 58 spent three times as much, 43 spent five times as much, and 27 spent ten times as much.[29] In contrast, spending on research and development in Canada exceeded that spent on promotion, although the authors acknowledged limitations on the data.[30]

Whatever the present costs of prescription drugs might be, the advent of personalized medicine, particularly drugs developed on the basis of one's genetic profile, will no doubt raise the costs significantly. Indeed, this was obvious even in 1998, when trastuzumab was approved for the treatment of breast cancer marked by high levels of human epidermal growth factor receptor 2, secondary to mutations in the BCR-ABL gene. At that point, the drug cost about $60,000 yearly,[31] while drugs aimed at Gaucher's disease and paroxysmal nocturnal hemoglobinuria cost about $300,000 yearly.[32] While these costs may not be precisely what patients are charged, someone has to pay! Certainly no one wishes to deny patients with these serious illnesses the best treatment; there are costs to society and the health care system[33] that need to be discussed. This could become even more urgent, should precision medicines for mental disorders be developed,[34] given the prevalence of depression, ADHD, and other illnesses, many of which have varying courses and different symptom presentations.

Yet another opportunity for Pharma has been the rise of advocacy groups for a variety of illnesses. These include the National Alliance for the Mentally Ill (NAMI), an organization that received $11 million from Pharma during the years 1996–1999,[35] with Eli Lilly contributing $1.1 million in 1999, and over $540,000 in 2007.[36] The money continued to roll in during the years 2006–2008, when NAMI received almost $23 million from Pharma, according to Gardner Harris.[37] This amounted to 75% of NAMI's income during that period. The Executive Director of NAMI, Michael Fitzpatrick, acknowledged that 75% was too high and would drop significantly by 2010, which indeed happened. Note that in 2009, NAMI hosted a dinner with tickets priced at $300, although a pharmaceutical company was the sponsor.[37] Finally, it should not surprise anyone when NAMI resisted efforts by the Veterans Administration to limit access to the new second generation antipsychotics secondary to their enormous costs and metabolic side effects.

Adding to the opportunities for Pharma is the remarkable increase in the diagnoses of individual mental disorders to speak of the overall growth of the DSM.[14] For example, the diagnosis of bipolar disorder in youth under age 20 rose 40-fold during the years, a 10-year period from 1994-1994-2002-2003.[38] This followed a revision in the criteria for juvenile bipolar disorder in 1994. Similarly, following a revision in the definition of autism in DSM-IV, the number of children with a diagnosis of autism rose from one in 500 to one in 90 a decade later.[39] Similar concerns have been noted by Horwitz and Wakefield with regard to anxiety,[40] and Moynihan and Cassels, who fear that Pharma is turning us all into patients,[41] a concern echoed by Allen Francis in 2013.[42]

Yet, another opportunity for Pharma has come in the shift to an additional emphasis on the risk of diseases vs the diseases themselves, as described by Aronowitz in his book, *Risky Medicine*.[43] A few examples: We now are focusing on prehypertension and prediabetes, as well as early psychotic states. Such conditions clearly enlarge the market for antihypertensives and medications such as oral antidiabetic and antipsychotic medications.

At this point, however, we should narrow the focus and begin to describe the factors that have an impact on clinicians as they attempt to find a path toward improving the assessment of the risk–benefit ratio, a critical step in minimizing the risks and maximizing the benefits of their recommendations for care, whether for medications or non-drug therapies. Let's begin by examining Pharma's payments—some call them bribes—to physicians.

# References

1. Starr, P. *The Social Transformation of American Medicine. The Rise of a Sovereign Profession and the Making of a Vast Industry.* Basic Books, Inc., Publishers, New York, 1982.
2. Shorter, E. *A History of Psychiatry. From the Era of the Asylum to the Age of Prozac.* John Wiley & Sons, Inc., New York, 1997.
3. Valenstein, ES. *Great and Desperate Cures. The Rise and Decline of Psychosurgery and Other Radical Treatments for Mental Illness.* Basic Books, Inc., New York, 1986.
4. Younkin, P. Making the market: how the American pharmaceutical industry transformed itself during the 1940s. *University of California at Berkeley,* 2008. http://www.irle.berkeley.eud/culture/papers/Younkin-Mar08.pdf
5. Magee, M. *Code Blue. Inside America's Medical Industrial Complex.* Atlantic Monthly Press, New York, 2019.
6. Healy, D. *The Creation of Psychopharmacology.* Harvard University Press, Cambridge, MA and London, England, 2002.
7. Posner, G. *Pharma. Greed, Lies, and the Poisoning of America.* Avid Reader Press, New York, 2020.
8. Dean, CE. *The Skeptical Professional's Guide to Psychiatry. On the Risks and Benefits of Antipsychotics, Antidepressants, Psychiatric Diagnoses, and Neuromania.* Routledge, Taylor & Francis, New York and London, 2021.
9. Menninger, K, et al. *The Vital Balance. The Life Process in Mental Health and Disease.* Viking Press, New York, 1963.
10. Dean, CE. The death of specificity in psychiatry: cheers or tears? *Perspectives in Biology and Medicine* 2012.
11. Dean, CE. Social inequality scientific inequality, and the future of mental illness. *Philosophy, Ethics, and Humanities in Medicine* 2017; 12 10. https://doi.org/10.1186/s1310-017-0052-x
12. Angell, M. *The Truth About the Drug Companies. How They Deceive Us and What to Do about It.* Random House, New York, 2004.
13. Blumenthal, D. Doctors and drug companies. *New England Journal of Medicine* 2004.
14. American Psychiatric Association: *Diagnostic and Statistical Manual of Mental Disorders,* 3rd Edition. American Psychiatric Association, Washington, DC, 1980. For a comprehensive history of the DSM-III, see Decker, HS. *The Making of DSM-III, a Diagnostic Manual's Conquest of American Psychiatry.* Oxford University Press, New York, 2013.
15. Feighner, JP, et al. Diagnostic criteria for use in psychiatric research. *Archives of General Psychiatry* 1972.
16. American Psychiatric Association. *Diagnostic and Statistical Manual of Mental Disorders.* American Psychiatric Association, Washington, DC, 1952.
17. Dean, CE. Diagnosis: the Achille's heel of biological psychiatry. *Minnesota Medicine* 1991.
18. Paris, J. *Overdiagnosis in Psychiatry. How Modern Psychiatry Has Lost Its Way While Creating a Diagnosis for All of Life's Misfortunes.* Oxford University Press, New York, 2015.

19. American Psychiatric Association: *Diagnostic and Statistical Manual of Mental Disorders*, 5th Edition. American Psychiatric Association, Arlington, VA, 2013.

20. Faust, D, et al. The empiricist and his new clothes: DSM-III in perspective. *American Journal of Psychiatry* 1986.

21. Follette, W, et al. Models of scientific progress and the role of theory in taxonomy development: a case study of the DSM. *Journal of Consulting and Clinical Psychology* 1996.

22. Insel, TR. The NIMH research domain criteria (RDoC): precision medicine for psychiatry. *American Journal of Psychiatry* 2014.

23. Zachar, P, et al. The aspirations for a paradigm shift in DSM-5: an oral history. *Journal of Nervous and Mental Disease* 2019.

24. Moses, IIIH, et al. The anatomy of medical research. US and international comparisons. *JAMA* 2015. https://doi.org/10.1001/jama.2014.15939

25. Canipe, C, et al. How drug company revenue is driven by price increases. *Wall Street Journal*, 2015. http://graphics.wsj.com/price-hike-2015?mod=djem10point

26. Dieleman, JL, et al. US spending on personal health care and public health, 1996–2014. *JAMA* 2016. https://doi.org/10.1001/jama.2016.16885

27. Alcabes, P. Medication nation. *American Scholar* 2016.

28. O'Brien, PL, et al. Off-label prescribing of psychotropic medication, 2005–2013: an examination of potential influences. *Psychiatric Services* 2017. https://doi.org/10.1176/appi.ps.201500482

29. The R&D Smokescreen. The prioritization of marketing & sales in the pharmaceutical industry. *Institute for Health and Socio-Economic Policy, version 1.1*, October 20, 2016.

30. Lexchin, JL. Pharmaceutical company spending on research and development and promotion in Canada, 2013–2016: a cohort analysis. *Journal of Pharmacy Policy Practice* 2018. https://doi.org/10.1186/s40545-018-0132-3

31. Waltz, E. GlaxoSmithKline cancer drug threatens Herceptin market. *Nature Biotechnology* 2008.

32. Pollack, A. Cutting dosage of costly drug spurs a debate. www.nytimes.com/2008/003/16.business/16Guacher.html. Accessed March 26, 2008.

33. Dean, CE. Personalized medicine: boon or budget-buster? *Annals of Pharmacotherapy* 2009. For a discussion of the paper, see Leeder JS, Spielberg SP. Personalized medicine: reality and reality checks. *Annals of Pharmacotherapy* 2009. www.theannals.com, https://doi.org/10.1345/aph.1M065.

34. Insel, TR. The NIMH Research Domain Criteria (RDoC) project: precision medicine comes to psychiatry. *American Journal of Psychiatry* 2014.

35. Silverstein, K. Prozac.org. *Mother Jones*, November/December 1999.

36. Johnson, A. Under criticism drug maker Lilly discloses funding. *Wall Street Journal* 2007.

37. Harris, G. Drug makers are advocacy group's biggest donors. *New York Times*, National Edition, October 22, 2009.

38. Moreno, C, et al. National trends in the outpatient diagnosis and treatment of bipolar disorders in youth. *Archives of General Psychiatry* 2007.

39. Scull, A *Psychiatry and Its Discontents*. University of California Press, 2019.

40. Horwitz, AV, et al. *All We Have to Fear: Psychiatry's Transformation of Natural Anxieties into Mental Disorders*. Oxford University Press, New York, 2012.

41. Moynihan, R, et al. *Selling Sickness: How the World's Biggest Pharmaceutical Companies Are Turning Us All into Patients*. Nation Books, New York, 2005.

42. Frances, A. *Saving Normal. An Insider's Revolt Against Out-of-Control Psychiatric Diagnoses, DSM-5, Big Pharma, and the Medicalization of Everyday Life*. William Morrow, New York, 2013.

43. Aronowitcz, R. *Risky Medicine. Our Quest to Cure Fear and Uncertainty*. University of Chicago Press, Chicago and London, 2015.

# 2

# Industry Payments to Physicians
## *Research and Education or Bribery?*

## Introduction

As we have seen, the development of psychotropic drugs helped fuel the growth of Pharma and its extraordinary profits.[1] For example, the FDA approval of chlorpromazine (Thorazine) in May of 1954 let to $75 million in profits 1 year later for the manufacturer, Smith, Kline, and French. In a brilliant decision, the company had purchased the North American rights to chlorpromazine. During the years 1954–1964, antipsychotics largely displaced lobotomies and electroconvulsive therapy (ECT), resulting in more humane care and a dramatic increase in profits.[1] In the late 1980s and early 1990s, the appearance of blockbuster drugs such as olanzapine (Zyprexa), fluoxetine (Prozac), and their many look-alike successors, further increased the profit level. This took place in the context of the growth of corporate medicine, marked by the appearance of multinational corporations selling health services for profit.[2-4] Taking note of these developments, the *British Journal of Psychiatry* in 2003 published a debate, with David Healy[5] arguing that academic psychiatry had put itself up for sale, while Michael Thase argued that it is not unethical or immoral to work for the industry. However, Thase stressed that the regulatory system depends on the integrity of individual investigators. Unfortunately, this was the weak link in Thase's argument, as we shall see.

Indeed, concerns over the surge of financial conflicts of interest (FCOIs) between physicians and Pharma, and their effects on education, patient care, and research,[2,3,6] led to the development of the Open Payments Program under Section 6002 of the Affordable Care Act.[7] The Open Payments Program mandated the reporting of funds paid by Pharma to physicians, a process administered by the Centers for Medicare & Medicaid Services (CMS).[8] CMSS gather the data and make it publicly available at https://openpaymentsdata.cms.gov. Rosenthal and Mello soon characterized the program as a sunlit disinfectant applied to payments by Pharma,[9] payments which had—and still have—the obvious goal of influencing the prescribing habits of physicians, and solidifying their embrace of the burgeoning drug market.

Unfortunately, the extra dose of sunlight appears to have had effect on Pharma and physicians. In 2015, 48% of the physicians in the United States received $2.4 billion in payments, of which *only $75 million was aimed at research*, while $544 million went to ownership interests.[10] The largest chunk, $1.8 billion, went to so-called general (non-research) payments, with 87% of that money going for food and beverages, and $484 million for license or royalty payments. While the mean payment per physician was only $201, surgeons received $6,879, and males received higher levels of payments than females in each specialty. While the $201 payment at first glance appears inconsequential, Dejong et al.[6] found in 2016 that recipients of even a single meal, set in the context of promoting a specific drug, went on to prescribe that drug at a statistically significantly higher rate than a similar agent. This held true for statins, ß-blockers, and antidepressants.

DOI: 10.1201/9781003267218-3

A 16-page study[11] published in 2019 found that medical marketing in the United States during the years 1997–2016 increased from $17.9 billion to $29.9 billion. During the same period, marketing aimed at health care professionals increased from $15.5 billion to $20.3 billion. Of that, $13.5 billion was spent on free samples, $979 million on fees paid for company-sponsored lectures and meals related to specific drugs, and $59 million for disease awareness campaigns. Payments to key opinion leaders (KOLs), who are among the leaders in their respective fields, accounted for about 33% of company marketing budgets. (As we shall see, KOLs are in demand as honorary authors for research studies.) This study[11] also cited data on direct-to-consumer marketing, but we will examine that data in a later chapter. The authors concluded that these figures are almost certainly underestimates, since Pharma's spending on coupons, rebates, and online promotion could not be obtained. In addition, the data can vary, depending on the source. We should note that payments to physician's assistants, nurse practitioners, pharmacists, and dieticians had not been included in the Open Payments Act, but will be included starting in 2022, no doubt adding more evidence of Pharma's generosity.

Nevertheless, we must ask if these well-intentioned regulatory moves have in fact alleviated the concerns over the Pharma-health care entanglements. For example, Kanter and Loewenstein in 2019[12] stressed that transparency is not a significant solution to the issues surrounding COI, but instead may be a simple, but politically expedient and low-cost remedy that actually prevents the implementation of more effective strategies.

Given the data just cited, I decided to explore the Web of Science database on July 25, 2020, for relevant studies published in 2018–2020.[13] What I found was truly alarming, not only in terms of the hundreds of studies, but the frequency of payments extended to physicians at the top of the medical hierarchy. For example, Wong et al.[14] reviewed the Open Payments program to obtain Pharma's payments to "top tier" physician-editors of 35 highly cited medical journals during the years 2013–2016, and, as a comparison group, physicians by specialty. The journals included those in general/internal medicine, neurology, general surgery, psychiatry, pediatrics, and emergency medicine. The authors chose the top five journals in each of the seven categories, using rankings supplied by the InCites Journal Citation reports.[15] The term "top tier" was applied to physician-editors designated as the editor-in-chief, and those with titles such as deputy, senior, or executive editors. However, the authors excluded assistant, consulting, and managing editors. Non-clinical editors, including statisticians, were also excluded. Payments were classified as general, non-research, direct research, and indirect research funding, described as payments to the editor's research institution or other entity where the physician was a principal investigator.

Remarkably, 63.7% of the 333 physician-editors received Pharma-associated payments of any kind during the 41-month period.[14] Yearly general payments went to 41.7% of physician-editors, direct research payments went to 5.7%, and indirect research funding went to 18%. The 3-year total for general (non-research) payments to physician-editors was $23,000,594, vs $829,824 for direct research, and $31,500,838 for indirect research. If we look at individual data, the *mean annual general payment to physician-editors was $55,157* (italics mine), while the annual payment for direct research was $14,558. The mean annual payment for indirect research funding was $175,282, a payment highly valued by departmental chairs and deans, and thus greatly beneficial to the awardee in terms of promotions and prestige. Not surprisingly, most of these payments were higher than those received by non-editor physicians within their specialties. We should note that the NIH had designated $5,000 as a threshold that would indicate the possibility of a serious financial interest, although Wong et al.,[14] could find no empirical data to support that figure.

The authors expressed surprise at the findings, since the ordinary view of journal editing is one of a non-commercial task based on science, but the payments extended to physician-editors must necessarily invite concerns over the potential for bias. This is deeply disturbing, given the power of journal editors to select studies for publication, select peer reviewers, and in general influence the aims of the journals they head. Wong et al.[14] further noted the lack of a standardized approach for the process by which journal editors deal with their financial COI, or how they establish policies regarding recusal. This seems to be another setting in which transparency is only one step in curbing potential bias, since acknowledging payments by Pharma is not necessarily evidence of a bias-free approach.

Equally disturbing is a 2020 study of the financial ties between Pharma and the leaders of professional medical associations (PMAs) across the 10 costliest disease areas in the United States and Pharma.[16] The diseases included heart disease, trauma, mental disorders, diabetes mellitus, osteoarthritis, cancer, chronic obstructive pulmonary disease and asthma, back problems, infectious diseases, and hypertension. Using the Open Payments database, the authors traced payments to 328 leaders of 10 influential medical associations, including the American College of Physicians, the American College of Cardiology, the American Psychiatric Association (APA), the American Society of Clinical Oncology, the American College of Rheumatology, and five others. Financial ties to Pharma were assessed in the year of leadership, in the 4 years before leadership, and in the year after membership in the respective boards.

Before proceeding, we should note that medical associations have long been important to health care systems in that they not only represent their members, but are actively involved in medical education and the production of treatment guidelines.[16] However, the authors noted a paucity of data with regard to the their ties with the industry, with the exception of a study in Japan[17] which found that 87% of board members of Japanese medical associations had received a total of $6.5 million from the industry. Moynihan et al.[16] also cited a U.S. study[18] that found general payments to 51% of medical journal editors, and research payments to 20%.

In the present study, Moynihan et al.[16] found that 72% of the 328 leaders had financial ties to the pharmaceutical industry, while 80% of the 293 leaders who were medical doctors or doctors of osteopathy had industry ties. Payments totaled $130 million for the 2017–2019 leadership, while the median payment for each leader reached $31, 805. However, the interquartile range was $1157 to $254, 272! Payments varied significantly, depending on the association, with only $212 going to the leaders of the APA, but $518, 000 to leaders of the American Society of Clinical Oncology. The authors emphasized that the very low payments to the APA indicate that medical associations can survive without strong financial ties to industry, although, as we have seen elsewhere, individual members of the APA are strongly tied to Pharma via consultancies, fees for lectures favorable to the product, and as patent holders.[19, pp.32–35] Nevertheless, this study, as well as the study on payments to journal editors,[14] provide strong evidence that editors and medical associations cannot claim independence from industry influence. Bias is everywhere!

## From bias to costs

The consequences of the physician-industry entanglement go well beyond bias, and clearly affect the costs of the United States health care system, the most expensive in the world.[20,21, p.2–3] For example, in 2019, Mejia et al.[22] linked 374,766 industry payments to providers with Medicare data on health care costs, after noting that the cost of drugs is among the largest drivers of costs in Medicare. (Indeed, drug costs have been a primary source of the differences in health-care costs when comparing the United States with other countries.[20]) In general, providers receiving higher payments from industry tended to bill higher drug and medical costs, with a significant association between payments and medical costs that extended well past the association between payments and drug costs. For an individual provider, a $25 difference in payments was associated with an $1,100 difference in annual Medicare medical costs, and a difference of $100 in drug costs. Interestingly, there was a stronger association between payments and medical costs in larger states with a more conservative political ideology.

With regard to transparency, the authors reinforced others who have noted that additional transparency has not reversed the links between Pharma and providers. Indeed, payments to providers increased from $4.3 billion in 2013 to $8.8 billion in 2016! The authors further noted that they did not divide payments into the usual categories of with research vs non-research general payments, and did not examine non-Medicare costs.[22] Nor could they establish a strict causal relationship between payments and costs, but reminded us that the AMA's Code of Ethics specifically notes that industry gifts create the risks of subtly biasing one's professional judgement in the care of patients."[23]

With regard to industry payments and the effects on Medicare Part D, Sharma et al.[24] linked data from the Open Payments database with data from the 2014 Medicare Part D Prescriber Public Use File. The focus was on 667,278 physicians who had prescribed one of six brand-name drugs, although each of the branded drugs had an equally effective but less costly alternative. The patterns described above continued to hold, with a higher odds of prescribing three of the six brand-name drugs among those physicians who had received industry payments. If payments had been made by the manufacturer of a specific brand-name drug, physicians were more likely to prescribe four of the six brand-name drugs.

Medicare Part D drug utilization data linked with the Open Payments database also revealed a disturbing association between industry payments and higher volume of opioid prescriptions in 2013–2015.[25] Unfortunately, prescriptions for opioids had more than tripled during the years 1999–2015, while rates of misuse and overdoses had increased. The authors also noted that prior studies had found links between opioid-related promotional activities and increased prescribing rates of opioids—never mind the epidemic. Given the need for additional research in this area, the authors developed two sets of physicians, one of which had received opioid-related payments in 2014–2015 but not in 2013, and another set where such payments were received in 2015, but not in 2013 or 2014. The primary outcomes focused on daily doses filled, expenditures per daily dose, and expenditures on filled prescriptions. Comparison groups had not received any opioid-related payments in any year. What were the results?

Those physicians receiving opioid-related payments had significantly increased opioid expenditures, daily doses dispensed, and higher expenditures per daily dose.[25] As with the studies noted earlier, higher payments were associated with larger increases in all three measures. Not only did payments result in an increase in prescriptions, but in a shift toward prescribing more expensive opioids. With regard to the size of payments, the mean total for the set of physicians prescribing in 2014–2015, was $251, and but only $40 for the set of physicians prescribing opioid only in 2015; nevertheless, this group also had increases in the three outcome measures, but less so than in the 2014–2015 group.

This data confirms the role of physicians in the opioid epidemic, a phenomenon explored in detail by Sam Quinones in his book, *Dreamland: The True Tale of America's Opiate Epidemic*,[26] a book I strongly recommend. There is little doubt that the manufacturers of opioids engaged in a campaign aimed at convincing health care providers that oxycontin was safe and minimally addictive, but we cannot explore that here.

Yet another area of interest is oncology, given the extraordinary costs of its drugs, and "… the dominance of oncology products in the global pharmaceutical market," as cited by Haque et al., in 2020.[27] That being the case, Haque et al. linked non-research industry payments obtained from the Open Payments database to 443 physician editors of 26 oncology research journals.[27] To be included, the journals must have published at least one interventional clinical trial. The authors noted that research payments from industry may well be necessary for advances in the treatment of cancer, but non-research payments could be eliminated without endangering new treatments. *Nevertheless, non-research payments were given to 80% of physician editors.* The mean payment per editor was $106,773; the median was $8,227, while 77% of journals had an editor whose payment was greater than $100,000! Editor-in-chiefs did even better, with a mean payment of $125,812, and a median payment of $22,308 In addition, the total value of payments increased from $1,732,240 in 2013 to $7,992,980 in 2018, a six-fold increase. Given these sums, did the editors acknowledge the value of their payments? Rarely. In fact, only five journals had posted COI accessible online. In three of the five, at least one editor reported no COI—despite receiving payments—a problem with 11 of 57 eligible editors.

The fact that non-research, general payments increased by such an extent, at least in oncology, is alarming. The lack of transparency is striking, and again reflects the failure of science to stem the influence of industry in academic medicine, despite multiple attempts to do so, as I will describe later.

But oncologists are not the only group affected by its relationship with industry. For example, payments by industry to neurologists in 2013–2015 were investigated by Robbins et al.,[28] using the Open Payments database. During that period, 1.6 million payments were made to at least 9,505 neurologists for a total of $354 million. Between 65% and 80% received less than $1,000 yearly, but at least 200 received over $100,000 during some years, and a few received over $1 million.

Although we have focused on general, non-research payments, past studies have examined the influence of corporate support with regard to grants and contracts,[29] but what about corporate gifts? Campbell and associates[30] examined this issue by mailing a survey to 3,300 faculty involved in life science research in the 50 universities that had received the most research funding from the NIH in 1993. Half of the faculty sample was derived from clinical departments ($n = 1,871$), half ($n = 1,871$) from non-clinical departments, and 258 from faculty that had received grants from the Human Genome Project.

Sixty-four percent responded to the survey,[30] with 43% reporting a research-related gifts independent of a research contract or grant. Of the 43%, 24% received biomaterials, 15% received discretionary funds, 11% research equipment and trips to meetings, 9% support for students, and 3%, other research-related gifts. Just over 50% received more than one type of gift. There was no difference in the percentage receiving gifts when comparing clinical vs non-clinical departments or if receiving Human Genome Project funding. However, more gifts went to senior and male faculty, a finding common in other studies.

It was clear that the gifts came with strings attached. Indeed, 63% reported that the donors expected acknowledgment in publications, while 43% said the gift was not to be used commercially or in competition with the company's products. Nineteen percent wanted ownership of any research that led to patents. Despite these requests and restrictions, 66% reported that the gifts were important to their research.[30] Unfortunately, the authors had no information from the recipients with regard to their compliance with limitations set by the donors, nor did they have any information on the dollar amounts of the gifts, data which would have been very interesting.

While several of the studies just reviewed indicated that payments to physicians had increased with time, one study in 2019 found a bright spot, with a decline in payments over time.[31] The author identified 409,000 physicians who had delivered Medicare services on an outpatient basis in 2014, and tracked their receipt of industry payments between 2014 and

2016. He also examined the Medicare Part D prescription behavior of 741,000 physicians between 2014 and 2015. Industry transfers were tracked in six categories: food and beverage, education, travel/lodging, fees for consulting, and compensation for other services. The author further stressed that prior studies had not included state controls, an important issue given the differences among states in reporting requirements and restrictions on physician-industry relationships.

This paper has an extraordinarily complex set of data, but the results are similar to other studies in that those who accept more industry payments are males with larger office-based practices and those with greater Medicare treatment volumes. However, the likelihood of payments declined substantially over the observation period.[31, p.646] Nevertheless, acceptance of payment transfers, or a higher number of transfers, led to higher prescription costs, more prescriptions for brand-name drugs, and higher rates of prescriptions involving high-risk drugs for older patients, a significant clinical issue.

## Conflicts of interest: Massive ambivalence in *JAMA*

The *Journal of the American Medical Association* (*JAMA*) devoted the May 2, 2017 issue (volume 317, number 17) to issues surrounding COIs. While I give credit to *JAMA* for the effort, which included several editorials and 23 Viewpoints,[32] a close reading indicates that the authors were awash in a sea of ambivalence! Taken as a whole, the imperative seemed be a search for how investigators can avoid serious COIs, but still maintain their close ties to industry and its wealth, wealth which was viewed as indispensable in the search for better treatment strategies. In a lengthy editorial,[32] the executive editor and editor-chief of *JAMA* specifically stressed the "…enormous and important resources that industry provides to clinical investigation, with industry funding for clinical research far exceeding that provided by the National Institutes of Health (NIH)." In addition, the relationship between academic medical centers, individual faculty, and industry, has become progressively more complex. The latter point was emphasized by Pizzo et al.,[33] who noted that academic medical centers over the past 10 years have become more businesslike, as a result of the purchase of community hospitals and the establishment of health care networks. Academic centers have been forced to compete for revenue and market share, and emphasize the commercialization of discoveries via the pursuit of intellectual property rights, royalties, and equity. Obviously, the lack of funding by the NIH has been a driver of these clinical and commercial efforts.[33]

The increasing pursuit of financial interests was also noted by Steven Nissen,[34] a leading critic of the health care industry, who nevertheless acknowledged that PMAs not only have an important role in education, but in the representation of the financial interests of their members. This necessarily involves political lobbying and influencing health care policy. He also listed the various means by which PMAs solicit funds from industry, including industry advertisements in medical journals. Unfortunately, he did not appear to have access to the Moynihan study[16] in 2020 that described a median payment of $31, 805 to leaders of PMAs.

With regard to the pervasiveness of COIs, we also find a number of inconsistencies in the *JAMA* commentaries. For example, in an editorial, Stead[35] wrote that every professional has COIs,[35] ranging from the personal (their reputation, promotions), or external (financial interests in a not-for-profit enterprise). On the other hand, he insisted that "few professionals are intentionally dishonest," a judgment similar to that of Pizzo et al.[33] who noted that the "vast majority" of physicians are not driven by financial interests—despite the data we just reviewed. Stead went on to state that COIs and COIs plus dishonesty are at opposite ends of the spectrum. This continuum seemed to minimize the results of the studies we've reviewed that found very significant financial gains accruing to PMA leaders and journal editors. Even if this group of top-tier physicians were to openly and consistently acknowledge their payments, would they be considered free of bias? The evidence suggests otherwise.

In addition, the suggestion that all physicians have COIs seems a blatant attempt to dilute the problem. Indeed, if all professionals have COIs, how can they be a serious threat to integrity? This is nonsense. However, Lichter, in another Viewpoint,[36] echoed Stead,[35] pointing to data from the Open Payments database showing that more than 800,000 physicians have been recipients of industry payments since 2013. Thus, the almost the entire medical profession has a relationship with industry. However, since a $10 dollar threshold is the basis for reporting, Lichter posited that disclosure has gone too far. However, he then cited data showing that the median annual value of payments from industry to 600,000 physicians was $156, ten times the threshold he used to critique the flood of disclosures. Like the other authors in this series, he neglected the high value of payments to the top tier of physicians, who as leaders and editors wield great deal of influence in setting policy goals and priorities for the health care system. Yet, as Pizzo et al., insisted,[33] payments from industry do not necessarily indicate COIs, while, according to Lichter,[36] the seminal issue is not COI, but bias.

Nevertheless, Jansen et al.[37] have raised another issue in that authors and presenters of scientific data are subject to mandatory disclosures of COIs, reviewers of abstracts of medical conferences and journal editors are not subject to the same rule. This includes members of editorial boards, who play a major role in accepting or declining a publication and editing for content and journal requirements. This being the case, Janssen et al. conducted the first general assessment[37] of the prevalence of COIs among the editorial board members of 5 leading spine journals, the magnitude of those COIs, and the relationships of the board members with the relevant medical device industry.

Seven hundred board members were identified representing 595 unique individuals from 41 countries, 75% of whom were spine surgeons. Potential COIs were found in 29% of editorial board members, likely an underestimate, since not all board members could be identified. Of the 210 wo reported a potential COI, 76% had a financial relationship with one of the six leading medical device companies, and 42% reported a financial relationship of more than $10,000. Note that the extent of COIs varied from 0% in South America to 100% in Asia, and 64% in North America.[37]

Despite the publicity surrounding these payments, Pharma and physician scientists continue to find additional strategies aimed at enhancing their financial status. For example, an investigation by *Science* of the NIH Loan Repayment Program (LRP)[38] found that close to a third of 182 clinical science ambassadors did not follow the program rules against some forms of industry funding of their work. However, the NIH has found fewer violators. We should note the good intentions of the LRP, in that it aims to keep promising investigators in academic careers, rather than taking jobs in industry or private practice. On the other hand, other tax-payer funded loan forgiveness plans are strictly policed, and sometimes require commitments to various government entities as a condition. Not so the LRP, which at times has allowed industry support via direct payments or research funding with no limits set on amounts. Indeed, in 2017 reversed its ban on payments from Pharma, thus a paradox in that LRP became a pipeline to ties with industry! In any case, the LRP has paid out almost $1.1 billion for new or renewal awards to investigators, including $72 million in fiscal year 2018.

In fairness, *Science* also stressed the complexity of a shifting set of rules, such that the program's director, in interviews, had to reverse herself on the facts, and changed the accounts of past rules at different times, making hard conclusions difficult. Several outside commentators have noted that the rules are often chaotic, and lack underlying principles, fertile ground for evasion.

Not one of the authors attempted to shed light on the conduct of Pharma itself, although several inveigh against unscrupulous actors.[33,39] One would imagine, given the collective belief that collaboration between physicians and industry is vital for progress in developing new treatments, that the medical profession would be interested in the ethics of its principal partner, but there was no sign of that in these essays. This seems odd, since, according to Public Citizen,[40] Pharma paid a total of $38.6 billion in criminal and civil penalties during the years 1991–2017. This is a large sum at first glance, but it pales in comparison to the $711 billion in net profits accumulated by the 11 largest global companies.

Perhaps those profits encouraged even more generous payments to physicians, as noted by ProPublica which updated its database in 2019,[41] and found that at least 2,500 physicians have taken in at least a half-million dollars each during the years 2014–2019 from Pharma and device makers. Indeed, more than 700 doctors received at least $1 million! Note that these figures do not include money aimed at research or royalties for inventions. In addition, during each year from 2014 to 2018, drug and medical device companies spent $2.1 and $2.2 billion in payments for doctors for speaking and consulting, as well as for meals, travel, and gifts. ProPublica also included a detailed list of the top 20 drugs with the most annual spending 2014–2018, a number of which are very costly: no surprise here.

It appears that the Open Payments data, often promoted as a brake on Pharma, has not been effective in curbing Pharma's payments.

## Sunshine and levels of trust

Finally, it appears that these struggles may have eroded trust in the medical profession. One of the *JAMA* contributors[42] noted that the role of physicians is lessened when trust is diminished, but then cited a Gallup poll demonstrating the nurses, pharmacists, and physicians are among the most trusted professions by the public. However, several studies cited by Kanter et al.,[43] have found lower levels of patient trust in their physicians following disclosure of payments by Pharma, but others have found increased levels of trust. That being the case, Kanter et al. obtained a nationally representative sample of 3,542 adults in the United States, and asked them to rate their levels of trust in their own physicians. This was done in two surveys, the first in September of 2014, just prior to the first public disclosures of industry payments, and again in September of 2016. The authors also compared the responses from Sunshine states (Massachusetts, Minnesota) that had earlier passed disclosure laws, vs non-Sunshine states. The response rates to the survey were fairly good, with 61.5% responding to the second wave. The mean age of respondents was 53 years, and 54% were females. Only 8% were non-Hispanic black; 76% were white.

Public disclosure of industry payments was associated with a 2.7% decline in the level of trust in one's own physician; this was statistically significant.[43] However, there were geographical differences, with results from the Northeastern sample failing to reach statistical significance. Note too that only 3% reported knowing whether their physicians had received payments, but public disclosure apparently spilled over to those physicians who had not received any payments. The authors noted that trust in physicians has been associated with treatment adherence, improved disease self-management, satisfaction with care, and the use of preventative services, so even a modest decline in trust could have adverse consequences. They recommended wider acknowledgment of physicians who do not receive payments, and, like other authors in the *JAMA* issue, emphasized the median annual payment of $201 in 2015. Once again, we must note the neglect of research indicating that even simple meals or other gifts are associated with increased medical costs and prescriptions for more expensive medications.[23]

Unfortunately, residency training programs have often been associated with gifts from Pharma, as was noted in 2007 when 56% of internal medicine residency training programs accepted support from industry.[44] (I still recall drug reps handing out free textbooks and lunches, among other swag.) However, industry involvement has slowed over time in response to legislation, ethical concerns, and publicity. In a recent review of this development, Medscape Medical New reported data showing that 64% of family medicine residencies were "pharma-free," banning gifts of food, gifts, and drug samples, as well as interactions with medical students/residents and industry sponsorship of activities.[44]

Let's now move on to examine direct-to-consumer advertising, its origins, costs, and impact.

# References

1. Starks, SL, et al. The making of contemporary American psychiatry, part 1: patients, treatments, and therapeutic rationales before and after World War II. *History of Psychology* 2005.
2. Relman, AS. The new medical-industrial complex. *New England Journal of Medicine* 1980.
3. Bittker, TE. The industrialization of American psychiatry. *American Journal of Psychiatry* 1985.
4. Levenson, AI. The growth of investor-owned psychiatric hospitals. *American Journal of Psychiatry* 1982.
5. Healy, D, Thase, ME. Is academic psychiatry for sale? In debate. *British Journal of Psychiatry* 2003.
6. Dejong, C, et al. Pharmaceutical industry-sponsored meals and physician prescribing patterns for Medicare beneficiaries. *JAMA Internal Medicine* 2016.
7. Patient Protection and Affordable Care Act. Public Law 111-148, 111th Congress, Section 6002 (2010). https://www.govinfo./content/pkg/PLAW-111publ148/pdf/PLAW111publ148.pdf
8. Centers for Medicare & Medicaid Services. Search Open Payments. Open payments website. https://openpaymentsdata.cms.gov
9. Rosenthal, MB, et al. Sunlight as disinfectant—new rules on disclosure of industry payments to physicians. *New England Journal of Medicine* 2013.
10. Tringale, KR, et al. Types and distribution of payments from industry to physicians in 2015. *JAMA* 2017. https://doi.org/10.1001/jama.2017
11. Schwartz, LM, et al. Medical marketing in the United States, 1997–2016. *JAMA* 2019. https://doi.org/10.1001/jama.2018.1920
12. Kanter, GP, et al. Evaluating open payments. *JAMA* 2019.
13. Web of Science database, accessed July 25, 2020.
14. Wong, VSS, et al. Industry payments to physician journal editors. *Public Library of Science One* 14(2): e0211495. https://doi.org/10.1371/journal.pone.0211495
15. Clarivate Analytics. *Clarivate Analytics—InCites.* http://clarivate.com/scientific-and-academic-research/research-evaluation/incites
16. Moynihan, R, et al. Financial ties between leaders of influential medical associations and industry: cross-sectional study. *British Medical Journal* 2020. http://dxdoi.org/10.1136/bmj.m1505
17. Saito, H, et al. Pharmaceutical company payments to executive board members of professional medical associations in Japan. *JAMA Internal Medicine* 2019.
18. Liu, JJ, et al. Payments by US pharmaceutical and medical device manufacturers to US medical journal editors: retrospective observational study. *British Medical Journal* 2017. https://doi.org/10.1136/bmj.j4619
19. Angell, M. Conflicts of interest. *Fall Newsletter, Physicians for a National Health Plan.* www.PNHP.org
20. Papanicolas, I, et al. Health care spending in the United States and other high-income countries. *JAMA* 2018.
21. Magee, MPSPCB. *Inside America's Medical Industrial Complex.* Atlantic Monthly Press, New York, 2019.

22. Mejia, J, et al. Open data on industry payments to healthcare providers reveal potential hidden costs to the public. *Nature Communications*. http://doi.org/10.1038/s41467-019-12317-z

23. Steinbrook, R. Physicians, industry payments for food and beverages, and drug prescribing. *JAMA* 2017.

24. Sharma, M, et al. Association between industry payments and prescribing costly medication: an observational study using open payments and Medicare Part D data. *BioMed Central Health Services Research* 2018. https://doi.org/10.1186/s12913-018-3043-8

25. Zezza, MA, et al. Payments from drug companies to physicians are associated with higher volume and more expensive opioid analgesic prescribing. *Public Library of Science One* 13(12): e0209383. https://doi.org/10.1371/journal.pone.0209383

26. Quinones, S. *Dreamland. The True Tale of America's Opiate Epidemic.* Bloomsbury Press, New York, 2015.

27. Haque, W, et al. Non-research pharmaceutical industry payments to oncology physician editors. *The Oncologist* 2020. http://dx.doi.org/10.1634/theoncologist.2019-0828

28. Robbins, NM, et al. Scope and nature of financial conflicts of interest between neurologists and industry. *Neurology* 2019. https://doi.org/10.1212/WNL.0000000000008067

29. Blumenthal, D, et al. Participation of life science faculty in research relationships with industry. *New England Journal of Medicine* 1996.

30. Campbell, EG, et al. Looking a gift horse in the mouth. Corporate gifts supporting life sciences research. *JAMA* 1998.

31. Brunt, CS. Physician characteristics, industry transfers, and pharmaceutical prescribing: empirical evidence from Medicare and the Physician Payment Sunshine Act. *Health Services Research* 2019. http://dx.doi.org/10.1111/1475-6773,13064

32. Fontanarosa, P, et al. Conflict of interest and medical journals. *JAMA* 2017.

33. Pizzo, PH, et al. Role of leaders in fostering meaningful collaborations between academic medical centers and industry while also managing individual and institutional conflicts of interest. *JAMA* 2017.

34. Nissen, SE. Conflicts of interest and professional medical associations. Progress and remaining challenges. *JAMA* 2017.

35. Stead, WW. The complex and multifaceted aspects of conflicts of interest. *JAMA* 2017.

36. Lichter, AS. Conflict of interest and the integrity of the medical profession. *JAMA* 2017.

37. Janssen, SJ, et al. Potential conflicts of interest of editorial board members of five leading spine journals. *Public Library of Science One* 2015.

38. Pillar, CDD. An NIH program repays school debt to keep scientists in academia. Many break the rules by also taking industry money. *Science* 2019.

39. Bero, L. Addressing bias and conflict of interest among biomedical researchers. *JAMA* 2017.

40. Twenty-seven years of pharmaceutical industry criminal and civil penalties: 1991-2017. March 14, 2018. https://citizen.org/sites/default/files/241.pdf

41. Ornstein, C, et al. We found over 700 doctors who were paid more than a million dollars by drug and medical device companies. *ProPublica*, October 17, 2019.

42. Fineberg, HV. Conflict of interest. Why does it matter? *JAMA* 2017.

43. Kanter, JP, Carpenter, D, Lehmann, LS, et al. US nationwide disclosure of industry payments and public trust in physicians. *JAMA Network Open* 2019. http://dx.doi.org/10.1001/jamanetworkopen.2019.1947

44. Ault, A. Family medicine residencies increasingly eschew pharma influence. *Medscape Medical News* 2021.

# 3

# Direct-to-Consumer Advertising
## *Origins, Extent, and Consequences*

## Introduction

While a great deal of attention has been devoted to direct-to-consumer advertising (DTCA) in recent years,[1,2] this is not a new phenomenon. Indeed, we need to return to the 17–19th centuries to see the roots of what is now a multi-billion dollar strategy by Pharma. However, the history of DTCA is marked by a no-holds barred approach to the development and sale of drugs. In the colonies, there were no boundaries between professionals and tradesmen, as Paul Starr[3] has emphasized. This was a period in which virtually anyone could self-identify as a physician, and legally advertise and sell his or her homemade remedies, often in addition to other services such as midwifery,[3, p.37] but, as mentioned earlier there was no regulatory oversight. Although the first law requiring an examination and certification of physicians was enacted in 1760, unlicensed (lay) doctors continued to increase,[3, p.44] as did the swamp of homemade remedies.

By the mid-19th century, a number of pharmaceutical companies had made their appearance, including Eli Lilly, Parke-Davis, Merck, and E.R. Squibb & Sons, several of which began to focus on cocaine and opiates. Heroin was marketed by Bayer in 1900 for use as a cough syrup, and as a treatment for schizophrenia, asthma, and seizures.[2, pp.6–10] Anyone over age 18 could buy it. No prescriptions were required for opiates, cocaine, or other toxic compounds, despite soaring rates of addiction. (It took another 19 years before prescriptions were mandated for the use of heroin.) In the meantime, hundreds of smaller firms selling a variety of patent medicines were still in action, selling some 50,000 homemade "miracle cures," all readily available in the marketplace. The larger drug companies found themselves in competition with the smaller firms, but even the smaller companies developed patent medicines that led to huge profits for the owners. As Posner noted,[2, p.8] the fight for money led to a deluge of advertisements in newspapers, billboards, and posters, touting the miraculous effects of elixirs made of alcohol, herbs, opium, and cocaine. Sales of these agents eventually reached $100 million yearly,[3, p.24] making it obvious that advertising was highly effective.

It was not until the early 1900s that serious questions were raised about the damage that the so-called miracle cures were inflicting on the population. Indeed, a long series of articles in Collier's magazine in 1905–1906 led to a reform movement that culminated in the Pure Food and Drug Act in 1907.[2, p.582–583] In 1905, *JAMA* published an editorial[4] decrying the misrepresentation and fraud perpetrated by the manufacturers of nostrums and the various miracle cures. The Proprietary Association of America also came under fire for its lobbying efforts.[2,p.584] In the meantime, bromides, barbiturates, and choral hydrate were mainstays in the

DOI: 10.1201/9781003267218-4

community. All were available without a prescription. It was not until the Humphrey-Durham amendments to the 1938 Food, Drug, and Cosmetic Act that prescriptions would be required for all new medications.[5, p.35]

# DTCA: A Success Story for Industry

The first 50 years of the 20th century witnessed the discovery of vitally important drugs, including insulin in 1922, penicillin in 1928, and sulfa drugs in the 1930s. At that point, attention turned to psychiatry, which had been busy developing electric shock therapy, insulin coma, and prefrontal lobotomies,[6] none of which lent themselves to massive advertising campaigns, but were widely used in the asylums. However, treatment of mental disorders was not a favorite subject in medical journals, and of little interest to Pharma. For example, the *British Journal of Psychiatry* in 1930 published only 5 articles on treatment, 3 in 1935, and 34 in 1940. Eighteen of the 34 focused on insulin coma.[7]

By 1950, electroshock and lobotomy dominated articles on treatment, but advances in drug therapy were only a few years away. The advent the mid-1950s of chlorpromazine, the first antipsychotic, and imipramine, the first antidepressant, contributed greatly to the wealth and power of Pharma, although companies had begun to increase their investment in research by 1945,[3,p.339] spending $40 million, almost twice the amount spent by foundations and universities. However, sales of antipsychotics and antidepressants provided a dramatic boost to their earnings. For example, after Smith, Kline, and French invested $350,000 in chlorpromazine, their sales steadily increased, rising from $53 million in 1953 to $347 million in 1970, of which $116 million was derived from sales of chlorpromazine.[8, p.155] With the development of risperidone and olanzapine in the mid-1990s, revenues increased even more dramatically, with risperidone bringing in over $500 million in 1996, and olanzapine over $1 billion in 1998. That same year, sales of antipsychotics in the United States reached $2.3 billion.[8, pp.260–261.]

Antidepressants were not far behind, with the discovery and marketing of imipramine in the late 1950s, followed quickly by amitriptyline and others. By 1980, ten million prescriptions for antidepressants were written in the United States alone,[9, p.261] but, with the marketing of fluoxetine (Prozac) in 1986, sales exploded, with Prozac becoming the second best-selling drug in the world in 1994, bringing in some $4 billion annually.[9, p.324]

The FDA handed Pharma another gift when in 1997 it lifted the restrictions on advertising of pharmaceuticals,[10] restrictions that began with a moratorium in 1983, but was partially reversed in 1995.[11] Pharma quickly began a series of marketing efforts, involving, for example, nicotine patches, leading to an $800 million market. Another DTCA campaign focused on Claritin, and resulted in the manufacturer capturing over half of the $1.8 billion market for non-sedating antihistamines.[12] These results were not lost on the industry. By 1997, spending on DTCA was $2 billion annually, increasing to $9.6 billion in 2016, with marketing aimed specifically at drugs growing from $1.3 billion to $6 billion annually, money that was spent on 4 million ads, including 600,000 commercials aired on television.[1] During the years 1999–2006, advertising led to a 300% return on investments made by Pharma.[13] We have already reviewed industry payments to physicians, but should add here that on average, Pharma was spending $61,000 per physician in 2004 on various forms of promotional activities,[1] including meals, trips, gifts, and company-sponsored "educational" events.

Given the data above, there is no doubt that DTCA was a stunning success for Pharma, but what about the effects on patients and prescribers?

# DTCA and Consumer Demand

At this point we can begin to explore the debate over the impact of DTCA. Friedberg and Bayer summarized the issues in 2017,[13] claiming that DTCA empowers patients in their quest to gain power in the usually one-sided physician-patient relationship. Proponents also claimed that DTCA not only provides patients with more information regarding medications and diseases, but enhances treatment adherence.[14] On the other hand, the opposition cited studies showing that DTCA provides inaccurate and misleading information,[14] damages the physician-patient relationship, drives up prescriptions for brand-name drugs, and significantly increases the cost of medical care in the United States. Indeed, Matthew Hollon[12, p384] concluded that the principal effect of DTCA marketing is to create consumer demand, while transforming the physician-patient relationship to a physician-consumer relationship. He also predicted that DTCA would expand its reach to the broadcast media, the internet, and would use web-derived data to target specific consumers with specific drugs—all of which occurred.

Indeed, the "patient as consumer" concept fits nicely with Paul Starr's concept of health care as a commodity,[3, p.22] as I mentioned in Chapter 1. In addition, we should note an emphasis in recent years on the creation of diseases by drug companies, as described by Moynihan and Cassels in their book, *Selling Sickness*,[15] and by Greenberg, in his volume, *The Book of Woe*.[16] Obviously, the business of creating disorders also involves physicians, who not only supply research into the pathophysiology of new disorders, but develop drugs aimed at their treatment.

With regard to patient demand, there is clear evidence that DTCA results in requests by patients for specific prescriptions, as shown in a review by Robinson et al., in 2004.[17] Indeed, 44% of patients received a requested drug in a study by the Kaiser Foundation,[18] while Lipsky and Taylor[19] reported that 71% of family physicians admitted that patient requests had pressured them into prescribing medications they would not ordinarily use. This was echoed in the survey done by Robinson et al.,[17] where 80% of Colorado physicians reported that patients had requested specific medications based on advertisements. They also noted that advertisements had lengthened the time spent in patient encounters, although one could argue that this is a positive effect, given the prevalence of the 20-minute med check. Colorado physicians also observed that advertisements did not provide good information on costs, alternative treatments and adverse events. Indeed, only 29% felt that DTCA was a positive development, but fewer than 25% believed that advertisements had actually changed their prescribing practices—in contrast to the findings of Lipsky and Taylor.[19]

These reports and studies clearly add another threat to balancing the risk–benefit ratio, no matter the field of medicine, and thus undermines the possibility of rational prescribing. This was demonstrated as well in a clever study by Kravitz et al.,[20] who created a randomized trial of standardized patients (SPs), e.g., actors portraying either a patient with symptoms commonly found in major depression, or a patient with an adjustment disorder accompanied by a depressed mood and low back pain. The SPs were seen as outpatients by internists and family physicians in four large physician collectives. The physicians were recruited by the authors, and were told only that they would be seeing two SPs several months apart. The SPs would present with common symptoms. Some of the SPs had been instructed to make a DTCA-driven request for Paxil (paroxetine) within the first ten minutes of the visit, or a general request for medication, or no explicit request at all.

Only 13% of physicians suspected that they had seen a SP, providing evidence for the reality of the encounters. In SPs with major depression, paroxetine was prescribed in only 3% unless

**25**

the SP specifically requested it. In that case, 27% of 51 requestors received it, while 26% received another antidepressant and 54% received no antidepressant. In SPs with adjustment disorder, antidepressants were prescribed in 34%, but 55% received an antidepressant if a specific request had been made. Prescriptions for paroxetine accounted for about two-thirds of all antidepressants given to those making a name-brand request in the adjustment disorder group. (There is no good evidence supporting a role for antidepressants in the treatment of adjustment disorders.) Overall, antidepressants were prescribed far more often when requested. Good follow-up care was provided for 98% of SPs in the major depression role who had made a general request, and in 90% of SPs who made a brand-specific request. However, only 56% of those making no request received adequate follow-up care, regardless of the diagnosis!

The authors conclusion: patient requests have a "profound" effect on physician prescribing when seeing patients with MDD and adjustment disorder.[20] This is obviously the case, but I am surprised that paroxetine was actually prescribed less frequently than other antidepressants in SPs making a brand-name request. On the other hand, prescriptions for antidepressants in the adjustment disorder group were clearly excessive.

Other studies have also shown that DTCA can lead to more demand and more prescriptions for a number of commonly used drugs, including those for asthma,[21] varinicline,[22] and antidepressants.[23] More recently, Layton et al.,[24] did an ecological study of over 17 million men in 75 market areas in the United States, using Nielson ratings for DTCA advertising of testosterone during the years 2009 to 2013. The Nielson ratings were then linked to data from commercial insurance claims. The main outcomes included rates of new serum testosterone levels, rates of initiation of testosterone use, and rates of testosterone initiation without using serum levels. To no one's surprise, exposure of unbranded advertising for "low T," resulted in increased rates of testing, new prescriptions for testosterone, and new prescriptions issued without testing. Interestingly, Pharma had begun to develop several new brands of testosterone, resulting in more branded advertising after 2012. Note as well a substantial geographic difference in rates of advertising, being highest in the Southeast and southern Great Lakes areas.

Each household exposure to advertising led to an increase in the three outcome measures, but the absolute rates were very low, at less than 1%.[24] In addition, the authors noted that the small, but significant increases in the outcome measures at 2 months, were lost in sensitivity analyses at 1 and 3 months. Nevertheless, we should emphasize that the use of testosterone had been FDA approved, but only for the treatment of hypogonadism secondary to changes in the pituitary-hypothalamic-gonadal axis. It had not been approved for decreases in testosterone or for non-specific symptoms in middle-aged or older males. In addition, several studies had raised concerns about the risk of cardiovascular adverse effects,[25] leading manufacturers to later discontinue DTCA for testosterone products.[24]

# DTCA and Patient-Physician Relationships

In a 2017 survey involving a representative sample of 1744 adults in the United States,[26] the authors explored how respondents viewed the impact of DTCA on their relationships with health care providers. (This relationship had last been studied by the FDA in 2002.) In this updated survey, 76% reported that they were likely to discuss an advertised drug with their provider, while 26% said they had already done so. Of the 26%, one-third asked the provider to prescribe the advertised drug, while 16% received it. This seemed unexpectedly low. Indeed, the authors pointed out that in the FDA survey of 2002, 49% had been given the requested advertised drug, so the drop in provider compliance appears to be a positive development.

On the other hand, 23% of respondents in the present survey[26] said they might switch providers if their provider refused to prescribe the requested drug, while 16% noted that advertising caused them to question their provider's advice. Only 5% felt that advertising had caused a conflict with a provider, which seems me at odds with the numbers suggesting they might switch providers, or had reason to question the provider's recommendations, based on advertising.

## Truth in Advertising: Should Consumers (Patients) Trust the Ads?

The FDA over the years has found many advertisements to be illegal due to the lack of information on adverse events and exaggeration of the benefits.[14] In 1999, for example, advertisements in magazines over a 10-year period did not supply information needed for an informed choice.[27] Similarly, DTCA ads on television in the years 2004–2007 associated the use of medicines with happiness and social approval,[28] a finding similar to my anecdotal observations that almost all DTCA television ads for oncology drugs portray cancer patients as highly energetic, bright-eyed, and difficult to distinguish from their non-afflicted friends or partners—despite the disease, and the graphic descriptions of side effects, including additional malignancies and other, possibly fatal, adverse events.

Advertisements in medical journals fared no better than DTCA advertisements. Indeed, this problem is not limited to the United States. For example, in a study[29] of six Spanish medical journals, the authors examined advertisements for antihypertensive and lipid-lowering drugs, and found that in 45 published claims of success, the promotional statements were not supported by the references. Similarly, Faeber and Kreling, in a content analysis of ads aired 2008–2010,[30] examined the most strongly emphasized claims of success in 84 prescription drug ads, and found that 55% were possibly misleading, and 2% were false.

## The FDA and DTCA

Before proceeding, we should take note of the FDA regulations pertaining to DTCA advertising. These regulations require a fair balance between risk and efficacy, regardless of the media.[10,11,31] However, the regulations for broadcast ads are somewhat less restrictive than for print, in that they are required to describe only the major risks, but these must be communicated in the audio. The risks must provide a source such that consumers can access the FDA labeling for the drug. The FDA does not approve promotions for off-label use. In fact, federal regulations ban DTCA ads from even suggesting off-label use, a requirement now under scrutiny by the Courts secondary to Pharma's claims regarding freedom of speech—an issue we will examine later.

Do the drug companies comply with these regulations and guidelines? Klara et al.[31] set out to examine the question, collecting all English-language broadcast ads aired in the United States from January 2015 to July 2016. They found 97 unique ads representing 60 unique drugs, and 67 unique drug indication combinations. Fifty-four ads were duplicates, so were excluded. None of the ads had information on the quantitative risks of the drugs. In contrast, 26% cited efficacy numbers. And, despite the ban on off-label promotions, *13% of the ads suggested off-label uses* for weight loss and reduction of blood pressure, particularly in drugs used to treat diabetes mellitus. The authors stressed that the quality of information presented in the ads was low, consistent with previous research on advertisements directed at both patients and prescribers, thus further muddying the risk–benefit ratio.

The FDA has not taken these failures lightly. As Parekh and Shrank have noted,[32] the FDA has succeeded in winning multiple lawsuits against Pharma for miscommunicating information in DTCA. In 2012 alone, GlaxoSmithKline paid out $3 billion and Abbott $1.6 billion in penalties. Three years earlier, Eli Lilly paid $1.4 billion, and Pfizer, $2.3 billion in settlements. As I pointed out in Chapter 2, Pharma incurred almost $40 billion in criminal and civil penalties during the years 1991–2017, but this was miniscule compared with $711 billion in net profits made by the 11 largest companies.[33]

Despite the fines and settlements, DTCA continues to expand. The U.S. Senate Committee on the Judiciary recently became concerned about the impact of DTCA on Medicare spending on prescription drugs, so requested and examination of the issue by the Government Accountability Office (GAO). The GAO report was issued in May 2021,[34] and summarized by Public Citizen in its newsletter, Worst Pills, Best Pills, in September 2021.[35]

During the years 2016–2018, Pharma spent about $18 billion in the United States on DCTA of more than 550 drugs, with $13 billion spent on television ads.[34,35] During that period, the Medicare program and its beneficiaries spent almost $324 billion on medications that had been the subject of DTCA, a sum that over half of the spending on medications under Medicare Parts B and D. The top ten drugs with the highest DTCA spending included three with the highest Part D spending: Humira, Lyrica, and Eliquis. One cancer drug, Keytruda had the highest Part B spending, and was one of the top ten in DTCA. Again, proof positive that DTCA is an effective strategy for Pharma. The Judiciary Committee responded by introducing a bill requiring that information on pricing be included in the ads.

# Patient Autonomy, the Internet, Telemedicine, and the Role of the Clinic

In recent decades, the traditional physician-patient relationship has been altered by the public's ready access to medical information on the internet and social media. Many patients arrive at the clinic having investigated their illnesses and treatment possibilities on the web.[34] Of course this includes DTCA, and easy access to direct-to-consumer laboratory testing. Depending on state laws, such testing can include comprehensive metabolic panels, complete blood counts, screening for hepatitis C, and screening for sexually transmitted diseases.[36] DTC genetic testing is more readily available, with the FDA in 2017 approving 23andMe's genetic tests that assess the risk for Alzheimer's disease, and nine other conditions. 23andMe then gained FDA approval for testing 3 BRCA1 and BRCA2 mutations involved in breast and ovarian cancer.[37]

In addition, Pharma's involvement with regard to social media continues to expand.[38] For example, Astra Zeneca set up a YouTube channel devoted to asthma, where it advertises its anti-asthma agent with videos and patient testimonials. Sanofi-Aventis also has a YouTube channel, "Go Insulin," using patient testimonials and informational videos, but omits the names of its insulin products. But You Tube isn't the only avenue for Pharma. Companies are also using Twitter accounts, blogs, and Apple iTunes.[39] Of course there are advantages to using social media for DTCA, including much lower costs than those found for branded advertisements, and the possibility of reaching millions of additional patients across the globe. This brings up another issue, since DTCA is legal only in the United States and New Zealand, but media advertising travels across boundaries. Spending for online marketing was estimated at $1 billion in 2010,[37] but is almost certainly much higher today.

The advent of direct-to-consumer telemedicine companies marks yet another phase in the delivery of health care services[40] that is well outside the usual clinic model. Jain et al.[38] list seven companies, three of which focus on erectile dysfunction and other genitourinary problems. Two focus on birth control, one on acne, and one on hair loss. In 2019, the companies raised an average of $66 million in venture capital, so the concept clearly is appealing, not only to investors, but potential patients, since the costs of prescribed drugs may be considerably lower, given the reduced overhead. Medical oversight varies considerably, ranging from a virtual visit with a physician for every patient, or, in some instances, a physician assistant or nurse practitioner. Others, especially the newer companies, offer medical contacts only to patients whose questionnaires reveal a contraindication to the requested drug. Obviously, this approach is not a comprehensive medical evaluation, and does not offer alternative treatments. Some companies state that they will send a report on the interaction to the patient's primary physician if requested. In addition, the FDA rules regarding off-label uses of drugs do not apply, so this opens additional possibilities for Pharma, with higher costs over time.

## Global Expansion for DTCA?

In 2008, *Psychiatric News*[41] reported pending legislation in the European Union (EU) that might allow some form of DTCA via print ads, television, and radio, although the proposal was not endorsed by the European Federation of Pharmaceutical Industries and Associations (EFPIA). Instead, the organization proposed an educational strategy focused on increasing information regarding diseases and how to prevent them, but without mentioning specific drugs. Naturally, PhRMA (the Pharmaceutical Research and Manufacturers of America) was all for global expansion. Indeed, Canada was also considering an amendment to the Canadian Food and Drugs Act that would allow DTCA via radio, print media, and television. Of course, a major problem to those who oppose globalization of DTCA is that the internet does not respect national boundaries. Whether this push for formal global recognition has succeeded is not clear. I have sent a request for information to EFPIA,[42] but as of August 2021, I have not received a reply.

## The Courts and DTCA

Here is another issue that could impact rational prescribing. As we have stressed, rational prescribing rests on balancing the risk–benefit ratio, a process that requires access to the relevant experimental data. But what if that data does not exist? What if the data exists, but cannot be accessed? This is relevant to the possible expansion of off-label prescribing which is legal in the United States, but, as noted previously, Pharma cannot promote drugs for off-label conditions, and the FDA does not require new data for off-label use. The prescriber is therefore free to prescribe a drug approved for use in schizophrenia to a patient with depression, despite the absence of new data. As one might imagine, Pharma is pushing to include off-label DTCA in its promotional activities, thereby expanding its sales and profits. Pharma has argued that the restrictions on off-label promotion violate the First Amendment. In 2015, a federal judge agreed, and ruled that the FDA could not restrict promotion of a company's fish oil drug.[43] The company, Amarin, had sued in Federal Court, claiming that it had the right to market the drug if a judge ruled that the marketing was not misleading or false.[44] In that case, marketing could proceed, even in the absence of proven benefits and FDA approval. In fact, the FDA had denied approval in 2013 for use of the fish oil drug in patients being treated with statins who had low levels of triglycerides, although it had been approved in 2012 for patients with very high levels of triglycerides. Kayczynski[44] also notes that a federal appeals court judge had cited *US vs Coronia*[45] in support of Amarin, and came close to declaring restrictions on off-label marketing unconstitutional. Interestingly, the decision on Coronia came only 3 years after the FDA sent warning letters to 14 pharmaceutical companies regarding the lack of relevant information in their online advertisements.[46] Did this data not matter to the court?

The debate continues, with Eguale et al.[47] describing multiple examples of adverse drug events associated with off-label prescribing in a study of 46,000 adult patients and 150,000 new prescriptions, with data gathered over 6 years. Unfortunately, fewer than 20% of the off-label prescriptions were backed by strong evidence. Patients receiving these drugs were almost 55% more likely to have an adverse drug event. In a review of this study, Good and Gellad[46] emphasize that clinicians often lack the time to assess the evidence behind off-label use, and thus may well lack the knowledge to accurately assess the risk–benefit ratio, making a balanced presentation to the patient difficult.

Even Thomas Stossel, who devotes an entire book to debunking what he calls the "conflict of interest narrative,"[49, p.xv] a movement he regards as having little if any merit, notes the possible adverse consequences of relaxing restrictions on off-label marketing.[49, p.224] Indeed, he calls for companies to do the hard work of developing clinical trials that would lead to FDA approvals—an excellent proposal, especially coming from an investigator at Harvard who admitted to an epiphany after being appointed to a Scientific Advisory Board at Biogen, where he became aware of the barriers encountered by those attempting to advance medicine.[49, p.xiv] Nevertheless, he admitted that the FDA assessments of product safety and efficacy "are the best analytical game in town."

Yet what we are now experiencing is an all-out effort to diminish the role of the FDA in its efforts to provide clinicians with the data necessary for balancing the risk–benefit ratio. The availability of biased and even outright false data on social media makes the role of the FDA even more valuable than in the past, so this is not the time for loosening restrictions on off-label use and enhancing the global reach of DTCA. Let's move on to other factors affecting rational prescribing, including publication bias, citation bias, and spin.

# References

1. Schwartz, LM, et al. Medical marketing in the United States, 1997–2016. *JAMA* 2019. https://doi.org/10.1001/jama2018.1920
2. Posner, G. *Pharma. Greed, Lies, and the Poisoning of America*. Avid Reader Press, New York, 2020.
3. Starr, P. *The Social Transformation of American Medicine. The Rise of a Sovereign Profession and the Making of a Vast Industry*. Basic Books, Inc., Publishers, New York, 1982.
4. Editorial. The power and influence of the Proprietary Association of America. *JAMA* 1905; XLV(21).
5. Healy, D. *The Creation of Psychopharmacology*. Harvard University Press, Cambridge, Massachusetts, London, England, 2002.
6. Valenstein, ES. *Great and Desperate Cures. The Rise and Decline of Psychosurgery and Other Radical Treatments for Mental Illness*. Basic Books, Inc., New York, 1986.
7. Moncrieff, J. An investigation into the precedents of modern drug treatment in psychiatry. *History of Psychiatry* 1999.
8. Whitaker, R. *Mad in America. Bad Science, Bad Medicine, and the Enduring Mistreatment of the Mentally Ill*. Perseus Publishing, Cambridge, MA, 2002.

9. Shorter, E. *A History of Psychiatry. From the Era of the Asylum to the Age of Prozac.* John Wiley & Sons, Inc., New York, 1997.

10. Food and Drug Administration. *Draft Guidance to Industry: Consumer-Directed Broadcast Advertisements.* National Press Office, Rockville, MD, 1997.

11. Food and Drug Administration. Direct-to-consumer advertising of prescription drugs: withdrawal of moratorium. *Federal Register.* September 9, 1985;50:36677–36678.

12. Hollon, MF. Direct-to-consumer marketing of prescription drugs. Creating consumer demand. *JAMA* 1999.

13. Friedberg, RD, et al. If it works for pills, can it work for skills? Direct-to-consumer social marketing of evidence-based psychological treatments. *Psychiatric Services* 2017.

14. Alves, TL, et al. Medicines, information and the regulation of the promotion of pharmaceuticals. *Science and Engineering Ethics* 2019.

15. Moynihan, R, et al. *Selling Sickness. How the World's Biggest Pharmaceutical Companies Are Turning Us All Into Patients.* Nation Books, New York, 2005.

16. Greenberg, G. *The Book of Woe. The DSM and the Unmaking of Psychiatry.* Blue Rider Press, New York, 2013.

17. Robinson, AR, et al. Direct-to-consumer advertising. Physician and public opinion and potential effects on the physician-patient relationship. *Archives of Internal Medicine* 2004.

18. Brodie, M. *Understanding the Effects of Direct-to-Consumer Prescription Drug Advertising.* Henry J Kaiser Family Foundation, Menlo Park, California, November 28, 2001. http://www.kff.org/content/2001/3197/DTC%20Ad@20Survey.pdf

19. Lipsky, MS, et al. The opinions and experiences of family physicians regarding direct-to-consumer advertising. *Journal of Family Practice* 1997.

20. Kravitz, RL, et al. Influence of patient requests for direct-to-consumer advertised antidepressants. A randomized controlled trial. *JAMA* 2005.

21. Daubresse, M, et al. Effect of direct-to-consumer advertising on asthma medication sales and health care use. *American Journal of Respiratory Critical Care Medicine* 2015.

22. Kim, Y, et al. Effects of televised direct-to-consumer advertising for varenicline on prescription dispensing in the United States. *Nicotine Tobacco Research* 2016.

23. Avery, RJ, et al. The impact of direct-to-consumer television and magazine advertising on antidepressant use. *Journal of Health Economics* 2012.

24. Layton, JB, et al. Association between direct-to-consumer advertising and testosterone testing and initiation in the United States, 2009–2013. *JAMA* https://doi.org/10.1001/jama.2016.21041

25. Finkle, WD, et al. Increased risk of non-fatal myocardial infarction following testosterone therapy in men. *Public Library of Science One* 2014.

26. Sullivan, HW, et al. Direct-to-consumer prescription drug advertising and patient-provider interactions. *Journal American Board of Family Medicine* 2020. https://doi.org/10.3122/jabfm.2020.02.19078

27. Bell, R, et al. Direct-to-consumer prescription drug advertising and the public. *Journal of General Internal Medicine* 1999.

28. Frosh, D, et al. Creating demand for prescription drugs: a content analysis of television direct-to-consumer advertising. *Annals of Family Medicine* 2007.

29. Villaneuva, P, et al. Accuracy of pharmaceutical advertisements in medical journals. *Lancet* 2003.

30. Faerber, AE, et al. Content analysis of misleading claims in television advertising for prescription and non-prescription drugs. *Journal of General Internal Medicine* 2013.

31. Klara, I, Kim, J, et al. Direct-to-consumer broadcast advertisements for pharmaceuticals: off-label promotion and adherence to FDA guidelines. *Journal of General Internal Medicine* 2017. https://doi.org/10.1007/s11606-017-4274-9

32. Parekh, N, et al. Dangers and opportunities of direct-to-consumer advertising. *Journal of General Internal Medicine* 2018. https://doi.org/10.1007/s11601-018-4329-9

33. Twenty-seven years of pharmaceutical industry criminal and civil penalties: 1991–2017. March 14, 2018. https://citizen.org/sites/default/files/241.pdf

34. United States Government Accountability Office. Report to Committee on the Judiciary, U.S. Senate: Prescription Drugs; Medicare Spending on Drugs with Direct-to-Consumer Advertising. May 2021. https://www.gao.gov/assets/gao-21-380.pdf. Accessed September 14, 2021.

35. Worst Pills, Best Pills. Direct-to-consumer advertising may be driving up Medicare drug spending. *Public Citizen* 2021.

36. Kilbride, MK, et al. The new age of patient autonomy. Implications for the patient-physician relationship. *JAMA* 2018. https://doi.org/10.101/jama.2018.1438210.1001/jama.5330

37. Gill, et al. Direct-to-consumer genetic testing: the implications of the US FDA's marketing authorization for BRCA testing. *JAMA* 2018. https://doi.org/10.1001/jama.5330

38. Yan, J. FDA catching up with companies that push online envelope. *Psychiatric News*. https://doi.org/10.1176/pn.44.6.0002

39. Liang, BA, et al. Direct-to-consumer advertising with interactive internet media. Global regulation and public health issues. *JAMA* 2011.

40. Jain, T, et al. Prescriptions on demand. The growth of direct-to-consumer telemedicine companies. *JAMA* 2019. https://doi.org/10.1001/jama.2018.19320

41. Yan, J. DTC advertising going global, but not without controversy. *Psychiatric News*, published online:16 May 2008. https://doi.org/10.1176/pn.43.10.0001a

42. Dean, C. Email to the European Federation of Pharmaceutical Industries and Associations, December 2020.

43. Johnson, C. FDA barred from restricting company's promotion of fish-oil drug. *Washington Post*. http://www.washingtonpost.com/news/wonkblog/wp2015/08/07/fda-barred-from-restricting-companys-promotion-of-fish-oil-drug/

44. Kapczynski, A. Free speech and pharmaceutical regulation—fishy business. *JAMA Internal Medicine* 2016. https://doi.org/10.1001/jamainternmed.2015.8155

45. U.S. v. Coronia, 703 f.3d 149 (2012).

46. Yan, J. FDA catching up with drug companies that push online envelope. *Psychiatric News*, published online: 5 June 2009. https://doi.org/10.1176/pn.44.11.oo4afty

47. Eguale, T, et al. Association of off-label drug use and adverse events in an adult population. *JAMA Internal Medicine*. 2015. https://doi.org/10.1001/jamainternmed.2015.6058

48. Good, CB, et al. Off-label drug use and adverse events. Turning up the heat on off-label prescribing. *JAMA Internal Medicine* 2016;176:63–64. https://doi.org/10.1001/jamainternmed.2015.6068

49. Stossel, TP. *Pharmaphobia. How the Conflict of Interest Myth Undermines American Medical Innovation*. Rowman & Littlefield, Lanham, BO, New York, London, 2015.

# 4

# Publication and Citation Bias, Spin, and Sponsorship
## Tilting the Risk–Benefit Ratio

## Introduction

Evidence-based medicine (EBM) has been a cornerstone of contemporary medicine for the past several decades. In 1959, EBM was defined[1, p.71] as a conscientious, explicit, and judicious use of current best evidence in making decisions about the care of individual patients, a process that necessarily underlies rational prescribing. Yet, in 2013, Steven Nissen of the Cleveland Clinic admitted that publication bias, particularly the failure to publish negative studies, continues to corrupt nearly every aspect of our profession.[2, p.671] The more colorful term: the file drawer problem. In his 2013 essay, Nissen went on to note[2, p.671] several of the more flagrant examples of publication bias, including the failure of the drug company selling rosiglitazone to publish 35 of 42 trials that sought to establish its cardiovascular risks. The full record became available only after litigation, as did the studies on the risk of suicide associated with antidepressant use in children. Nissen's concerns were not new: witness an article in 1959 that emphasized the likelihood of non-publication of trials with negative, or uninteresting results,[3] but, for all these concerns, an editorial in *Psychological Medicine* published in the year 2000 noted the lack relevant studies in psychiatry.[4] However, that deficiency has been corrected, as we shall see.

## Medical Research and Publication Bias

Before examining specific fields, what is the evidence for bias in clinical research generally? A 1991 study[5] in the *Lancet* examined 487 research projects that had been approved by the Central Oxford Research Ethics Committee in 1984–1987, and found 285 studies, 52% of which had been published. Studies with statistically significant results were more than twice as likely to be published (adjusted odds ratio of 2.32; 95% CI, 1.25–4.28). Fortunately, randomized clinical trials (RCTs) were less likely to be biased than were observational, and laboratory-based experimental studies, which were over three times as likely to be biased. Those studies with statistically significant results were also more likely to result in more publications, more presentations, and publication in journals with a higher-impact factor.

A narrative review[6] in 2010 came to similar conclusions with regard to publication of positive studies in higher-impact journals, faster publication, higher rates of covert duplicate publications, higher rates of citations, and the greater likelihood of publication in English. The authors also found evidence of reporting bias across 50 different diagnostic, pharmacological, surgical, and preventive strategies, so emphasized that the data indicated a widespread phenomenon in the medical literature that overestimated efficacy and underestimated risks.[6, abstract]

On the other hand, Fanelli et al., in a study[7] of bias-related patterns and risk factors in a random sample of meta-analyses taken from all disciplines, found that the magnitude of biases was rather small, although it varied widely across fields. It appeared that early, smaller, and highly cited studies were more likely to overestimate effects, as did studies by early career investigators, especially those working in isolation. Male and female investigators did not differ in their rates of bias, nor was there evidence linking bias to productivity. These patterns demonstrated modest increases over time, yet, in contrast to the many studies we shall review, the authors concluded that the scientific enterprise is not in jeopardy.[7, p. 3718] Nevertheless, such patterns need to be kept in mind when reading the literature.

Citation bias is a closely related problem, as one would expect, given the frequency of publication bias. However, Jannot et al.[8] point to studies from 2002 to 2007 that found citation bias in a limited number of topics. That being the case, the authors went on to examine all therapeutic interventions included in a series of meta-analytic studies in the Cochrane database published over a 3-month period in 2010. The goal: to determine if citation bias was widespread. The interventions were linked to citation counts in the ISI Web of Knowledge. They identified 89 research questions in 458 eligible studies, including those focused on infectious disease, cancer, cardiovascular disease, neurology, psychiatry, and others. Not surprisingly, the authors found that statistically significant articles were cited twice as often as non-significant studies, although the overall bias was labeled as "moderate." One important factor: significant studies were more often published in high-impact journals, a finding similar to those just reviewed. The authors also noted studies indicating additional associations with citation bias, including study length, number of co-authors, online availability, confirmatory bias, and attentional bias, wherein authors tended to recall statistically significant studies more readily.

Let's now move to more specific areas of interest with regard to biases in various fields, including oncology, depression, social sciences, drug trials, and others.

# Drug Trials: Background, Bias, and Negative Trials

Companies seeking FDA approval for new drugs (new molecular entities, or NMEs) must submit all trials, whether published or not, to the FDA as part of a new drug application (NDA). However, as Rising et al., have noted,[9] several early studies found selective reporting of trials and results. The authors therefore did a study[9] of all efficacy trials found in the NDAs and all published clinical trials related to the efficacy trials. The final sample included 164 efficacy trials related to 33 NDAs. Each published trial was assessed for design characteristics, funding, disclosure of conflicts of interest, impact factor, etc.

Critical questions: Are there discrepancies between trial data submitted to the FDA and data found in the published trials? Are there differences in the study characteristics reported to the FDA and in publications? Before answering these questions, I must stress that there was a significant problem with trial methodology, in that only 14% of the 164 trials used an intent-to-treat analysis (ITT) as the primary analysis.[9] What does this mean? An ITT analysis is preferable, since this includes all patients who began the trial, giving readers a more complete picture of the outcome. In contrast, a completer analysis gives the reader data only on those subjects who completed the trial, thus biasing the outcome.

With regard to the questions posed above, 78% (128/164) of the efficacy trials reviewed by the FDA were published, but, in a multivariate model, trials with favorable outcomes were almost five times more likely to published, while trials with active controls were three times more likely to be published.[9] Thirty-six trials were not published, but 15 of these were incompletely published in abstracts or a pooled publication. Twelve were verified as not published, while the authors could not determine what happened with nine studies, despite many contacts with the companies and authors.

Trials had a total of 179 primary outcomes reported in the NDAs, but forty-one of these were not to be found in the publications. Overall, the papers had more outcomes favoring the test drug than were found in the NDAs. There were 43 outcomes that did not favor the test drug in the NDAs, but almost half of these were not included in the published papers! Similarly, there were 99 conclusions in the papers and the NDAs. Of these, 10 did not favor the test drug, but, in 9 of the ten, conclusions in the papers reversed the conclusion reported in the NDAs, so now favored the test drug! In a detailed comparison of the NDAs and publications, the authors found multiple changes in the data on $p$ values, confidence intervals, and the frequency of adverse events, once again biasing the results.

The conclusion: the authors found substantial evidence of selective reporting of data and publication bias, indicating that publication of trial data in peer-reviewed journals is not adequately reported, is not complete, and likely biased in favor of positive outcomes. The authors also pointed to past studies showing that the failure to publish negative studies often stems from decisions by the investigators not to submit the data in publications, an issue I will take up later, since there are other factors at work.

The problem of negative trials also drew the attention of the *New York Times*,[10] where Aaron Carroll devoted an essay stressing the results of a number of studies in which primary outcomes were changed, results were spun in a positive direction, negative trials ignored, and the primary outcome was replaced with a secondary outcome, often without acknowledgment. Let's now explore some of these studies in more detail, starting with studies on depression and its treatment.

# Depression, Antidepressants, and Psychotherapy

In 2008, Erick Turner and colleagues published a seminal study[11] on publication bias in antidepressant trials, using data on drug efficacy gathered from published papers, and then comparing that data with data obtained from the required FDA reviews. The 74 FDA reviews covered 12 antidepressants ranging from bupropion to venlafaxine in studies that involved 12,564 adult patients. The FDA reviews were then matched to randomized, controlled trials in journal articles on the same antidepressants.

Interestingly, 31% of the FDA-registered studies had not been published. Why? It depended on the outcome, with 37 studies seen by the FDA as positive being published. Only one positive study was not published. In contrast, had the FDA found negative or questionable results, only 3 were published, while 22 were either not published, or spun in such a way that they conveyed a positive outcome! From another perspective, the published studies asserted that 94% of the trials were positive, while the FDA data indicated that only 51% were positive! The authors also noted that the effect sizes in the journal articles were always higher compared vs the FDA effect sizes, with the differences ranging from 11% (paroxetine CR) to 69% (nefazodone). Overall, the effects sizes increased by 32% in the published articles, clearly biasing the results in favor of the company's drug, and again tilting the risk–benefit ratio.

In 2017, de Vries et al. built[12] on the Turner et al. study[11] by adding 31 trials of novel anti-depressants approved after 2008, for a total of 105 depression trials. The results were similar, in that 98% of the trials considered positive by the FDA were published, in marked contrast to the negative trials, of which only 48% were published. A total of 77 trials were published, of which 32% were negative. However, 10 negative trials became positive in their publications, largely accomplished by switching the primary and secondary outcomes, or omitting unfavorable outcomes. Making matters worse, only 5% of the published trials "unambiguously" noted that treatment was not more effective than placebo.[12, p.2454] Consistent with other studies, positive trials were cited three times as often in the Web of Science a were negative trials.

Similar results were found by Roest et al.,[13] in a 2015 comparison of published RCTs vs FDA reviews of nine second-generation antidepressants used in the treatment of anxiety disorders, including panic disorder, social anxiety disorder, PTSD, obsessive-compulsive disorder, and generalized anxiety disorder. The drugs included paroxetine in several forms, escitalopram, duloxetine, venlafaxine in several forms, fluvoxamine, and sertraline. The authors found 57 FDA-registered trials, and 48 publications representing 52 trials, so performed a meta-analysis of both data sources.

Consistent with the Turner et al. study,[11] the FDA noted that 72% (41 of 57) of the trials were positive, but the journal articles claimed that 96% (43 of 45) were positive. Positive trials were five times more likely to be published, while the pooled effect size gathered from the journal articles was 15% higher that the effect size in the FDA data. However, the difference in effect size was not statistically significant, in contrast to the Turner et al. study.[11] Spin was found in 19% (3 of 16) of the not-positive trials, but was not present in the positive trials. The 3 articles with spin did acknowledge that the primary outcome was non-significant in their discussions of results, but claimed favorable results in the abstract, a strategy we shall note in other studies. (*This is a reminder that reading abstracts and conclusions may save time, but may be misleading.*) Despite the various forms of bias in this study, the authors concluded that biases, including spin, did not significantly inflate drug efficacy.[13]

Unfortunately, spin is not rare. In a much larger study[14] of 616 published reports of RCTs, 72 were ultimately identified as suitable for an analysis of spin, defined as an effort to stress positive results. These reports had clearly identified non-statistically significant results on the primary outcome measure. (Many of the 616 RCTS were rejected due to various methodological problems or were noninferiority trials, crossover trials, phase 2 trials, etc.) Spin occurred in multiple sections of the articles, to wit:

- In the title: 18%
- In the abstract under results and conclusions: 27% and 58%, respectively
- Main text results: 29%
- Main text discussion: 43%
- Main text conclusions: 50%
- Spin in at least two in the body of the main text: 40%

The authors also examined the maneuvers used in the attempts to make the outcomes more favorable. The most common approach involved emphasizing data obtained from sources other than the primary outcomes. These included secondary outcomes, subgroup analyses, or within-group comparisons. While subgroup analyses, when done openly, can lead to clues about drug effects in smaller populations, this was not the case in these studies. The authors stated that they could not identify the motives behind spinning, nor its effects on practice, but noted that reviewers and editors must be more vigilant with regard to such strategies, given the frequency of spin—especially in abstracts, on which busy clinicians often focus.

Publication bias also affects the data on efficacy of psychological treatments of major depression. For example, a 2010 study[15] comparing the efficacy of cognitive-behavioral therapy and other psychological approaches in 117 published trials, found evidence of 51 missing studies. After imputing results from the missing studies, the over-all effect size significantly decreased from 0.67 to 0.42, a 37% drop. However, Driessen et al.,[16] noted a methodological issue in that study, so decided that a more complete study of published and unpublished studies might be more informative. Driessen and colleagues,[16] therefore undertook a systematic review and meta-analysis of the U.S. National Institutes of Health-funded grants aimed at comparing psychological treatments vs control conditions for major depressive disorder during the years 1972–2008. They included some 30 different forms of psychological treatment, including studies of psychological therapies combined with an antidepressant or medication alone. Studies on maintenance therapy and prevention were excluded. The sole outcome measure was the severity of depression.

Interestingly, of some 4,000 grants, 3,841 were excluded, and others were excluded after not meeting DSM criteria for major depression, leaving 51 grants for the analysis. The literature search yielded 42 published studies and 11 unpublished studies. Of the funded grants, 23.6% did not result in publication, while two grant recipients never began a study. The addition of unpublished studies to published studies reduced the effect size from $g = 0.52$ to $g = 0.39$, a 25% drop in efficacy, fairly close to that reported by Cuijpers et al.[15] The authors concluded that psychological therapies for major depression are effective but that the effect size has been overestimated.

## Sponsorship and bias

Yet, in another perspective on bias and adult depression, Cristea et al.[17] in 2017 noted that the possibility of sponsorship bias in comparisons of the efficacy of antidepressants and psychotherapy had not been investigated for any mental disorder. Given the potential for bias secondary to sponsorship, they began a study of industry funding and conflicts of interest in authors who had published RCTs of pharmacotherapy and psychotherapy in adult depression. They excluded studies on maintenance therapy, but did not exclude studies with comorbid disorders, whether mental or somatic, an issue not addressed in the studies just cited. The final sample included 45 studies, 9 of which included comparisons between a form of psychotherapy and medication. Twenty studies had received pharmaceutical company support, while 21 did not.

After sensitivity analysis, trials without industry support failed to reveal any significant differences between medication and psychological therapies. Studies with industry support demonstrated a small but significant difference favoring medication in those studies with a low risk of bias. This finding was not unexpected, given studies cited by the authors showing that psychotherapy has been effective in treating adult depression. With regard to the authors' conflicts of interest, five authors had not reported financial conflicts of interest, although it was judged to be present. Yet studies wherein one or more of the authors had ties to the industry resulted in a small advantage of medication, but did not quite reach statistical significance. The authors recommended that authors reveal all industry ties, regardless of their relevance to the study at hand.

In contrast to this somewhat reassuring report, an analysis[18] of 319 randomized, controlled trials found that 182 had been industry-sponsored, and were 2.8 times more likely to report favorable results than did those without industry sponsorship. Studies with favorable results were cited more frequently, were larger, and were more frequently registered, a positive development. However, those trials were more often marked by non-inferiority/equivalence designs, meaning that the company goal was to demonstrate that its new drug was essentially equivalent to an established drug, rather than superior. (This has been very common in psychiatry, with the flood of "me-too drugs" dating to the 1960s.) Indeed, 96% of non-inferiority studies obtained favorable results, but what does this do for patients? Unfortunately, they do not represent any major therapeutic advances, and the new drugs are almost always more expensive.

The sponsorship problem is not limited to psychiatry. For example, a study[19] of 110 RCTs in three major neurosurgical journals in North America found that 78% of industry-funded trials had favorable results, vs 13% of those without industry sponsorship, a highly significant difference. Ivanov et al.[20] also examined three high-impact medicine journals in an examination of RCTs over three decades (1988–2008) in order to ascertain trends in publication. During those 30 years, the number of industry-funded trials doubled from 17% to 40%, while government-funded trials remained constant. It would seem that the marked rise in industry sponsorship would adversely affect the publication of negative trials, but it did not. In fact, the number of studies with negative results doubled from 10% to 22%, a significant finding, while lack of funding disclosure fell from 35% of trials to 7%. These are positive developments, but we should keep in mind the very poor results in 1988. Even with the changes, only 22% of the studies in 2008 were negative—still a low number. Nevertheless, another study[21] of 416 interventions and 360 RCTs in high-impact medical and surgical journals also failed to show an effect of industry sponsorship on the results of primary outcomes. Industry sponsorship was more commonly found in specialty journals, where it was strongly associated with trials of devices and drugs, but did not have an impact on primary or surrogate outcomes.

On the other hand, questions have been raised about the consistency with which clinical trials report funding, as noted by Hakoum et al.[22] The authors examined 200 RCTs published in 2015 in any of 119 journals. Of the 200 RCTs, 96% were funded, but the amount of funding was reported in only 1%, while the role of the funders was reported in 50%. Indeed, 42% of the funders were involved in study design and data analysis, and 41% in interpretation and trial management. This raises serious questions about the influence of funding agencies.

Although we have just reviewed several studies noting that the impact of industry funding may not be as significant as sometimes reported, Fabbri et al.[23] remind us that the industry has its own priorities, and thus focuses on products and activities that can be commercialized. Internal company documents have revealed the strategies used by industry to "reshape entire fields of research," and thus shift research agendas away from matters important to public health. We also have an updated Cochrane Review[24] that compared outcomes and risks of biases in studies funded by industry to studies without industry support. Both drugs and devices were examined in 48 controlled studies. Industry-funded studies had a 24% higher rate of favorable results and a 31% higher rate of favorable conclusions. With regard to drug or device harms, industry sponsored studies claimed an 87% decrease in harms vs non-industry funded studies. However, the data on devices is less certain than the data on drugs. The author also noted that Cochrane Reviews have not consistently examined industry sponsorship as a source of bias, a regrettable oversight.

Finally, Marcia Angell has provided multiple examples of the negative effects of our involvement with industry in an essay in the *New York Review of Books*, titled "Drug Companies & Doctors: A Story of Corruption."[25] This essay supplies references to a number of books and articles on the subject, and is well worth reading. But let's move on to a story of guests and ghosts, or how authorship is manipulated to enhance the value of one's work.

# References

1. Sackett, DL, et al. Evidence-based medicine: what it is and what it isn't. *British Medical Journal* 1996.
2. Nissen, SE. Biomarkers in cardiovascular medicine. The shame of publication bias. *JAMA Internal Medicine* 2013.
3. Sterling, TD. Publication decisions and their possible effects on inferences drawn tests of significance—or vice versa. *American Statistical Association Journal* 1959.
4. Gilbody, SM, et al. Publication bias and the integrity of psychiatry research. *Psychological Medicine* 2000.
5. Easterbrook, PJ, et al. Publication bias in clinical research. *Lancet* 1991. https://doi.org/10.1016/0140-6736(91)9021-Y
6. McGauran, N, et al. Reporting bias in the medical literature—a narrative review. *Trials* 2010. http://www.trialsjournal.com/content/11/1/37
7. Fanelli, D, et al. Meta-assessment of bias in science. *Proceedings of the National Academy of Science* 2017. www.pnas.org/cgi/doi/10.1073/pnas.1618569114
8. Jannot, A-S, et al. Citation bias favoring statistically significant studies was present in medical research. *Journal of Clinical Epidemiology* 2013. http://dx.doi.org/10.1016/j.clinepi.2012.09.015
9. Rising, K, Bachetti, P, Bero, L. Reporting bias in drug trials submitted to the Food and Drug Administration: Review of publication and presentation. *Public Library of Science* 2008. http://dx.doi.org/10.1371/journal.pmed.0050217
10. Carroll, A. Congratulations. Your study went nowhere. *New York Times*, September 24, 2018. https:www.nytimes.com/2018/09/24/upshot/publication-bias-threat-to-science.html
11. Turner, EH, et al. Selective publication of antidepressant trials and its influence on apparent efficacy. *New England Journal of Medicine* 2008.
12. De Vries, YA, et al. The cumulative effect of reporting and citation biases on the apparent efficacy of treatments: the case of depression. *Psychological Medicine* 2017. https://doi.org./10.1017/S0033291718001873
13. Roest, AM, et al. Reporting bias in clinical trials investigating the efficacy of second-generation antidepressants in the treatment of anxiety disorders. A report of 2 meta-analyses. *JAMA Psychiatry* 2015. http://dx.doi.org/10.1001/jamapsychiatry.2015.15
14. Boutron, I, et al. Reporting and interpretation of randomized controlled trials with statistically nonsignificant results for primary outcomes. *JAMA* 2010.
15. Cuijpers, P, et al. Efficacy of cognitive behavioural therapy and other psychological treatments for adult depression: meta-analytic study of publication bias. *British Journal of Psychiatry* 2010.
16. Driessen, E, et al. Does publication bias inflate the apparent efficacy of psychological treatment for major depressive disorder? A systematic review and meta-analysis of US National Institutes of Health-funded trials. *Public Library of Science ONE*. https://doi.org/10.1371/journal.pone.0137864.
17. Cristea, IA, et al. Sponsorship bias in the comparative efficacy of psychotherapy and pharmacotherapy for adult depression: meta-analysis. *British Journal of Psychiatry* 2017. http://dx.doi.org/10.1192/bjp.bp.115.17927
18. Flacco, ME, et al. Head-to-head randomized trials are mostly industry-sponsored and almost always favor the industry sponsor. *Journal of Clinical Epidemiology* 2015.
19. Khan, NR, et al. A review of industry funding in randomized controlled trials published in the neurosurgical literature-the elephant in the room. [Review] *Neurosurgery* 2018.
20. Ivanov, A, et al. Review and analysis of publication trends over three decades in three high impact journals. *Public Library of Science One* 2017.
21. Grey, P, et al. Outcomes, interventions and funding in randomized research published in high impact journals. *BMC* 2018. https://doi.org/10.1186/s13063-018-2978-8
22. Hakoum, MB, et al. Characteristics of funding of clinical trials: cross-sectional survey and proposed guidance. *British Medical Journal Open* 2017.

23. Fabbri, A, et al. The influence of industry sponsorship on the research agenda: a scoping review. *American Journal of Public Health* 2018.

24. Bero, L. Industry sponsorship and research outcome. A Cochrane Review. *JAMA Internal Medicine* 2013.

25. Angell, M. Drug companies and doctors: a story of corruption. *New York Review of Books*, Volume 56 Number 1, January 15, 2009.

# 5

# Fraudulent Authorship
## Ghosts, Guests, and Honorary Authors

## Introduction

We have focused thus far on a number of strategies used by Pharma to maximize profits, and by physicians to maximize their wealth, but these goals can also be enhanced via more subtle tactics. One of these involves manipulation of authorship, which can involve several different approaches. Let's first attempt to define the types of fraudulent authorship, but we should note that the definitions may vary, depending on the field and the journal.[1] In addition, studies have shown that expectations regarding disclosure of authors and their roles in research have varied not only across disciplines, but across cultures internationally.[2] Nevertheless, here are some common definitions.

*Ghost author*: A person who has been omitted from the authorship list despite qualifying for inclusion. Examples: employees of a drug company or device manufacturer, and medical writers employed by communication companies.

*Guest author*: A person who has not made a qualifying contribution to the study, but who may bolster the chance of obtaining a grant or acceptance by a journal.

*Honorary author*: A person whose inclusion as an author rests solely on his/her status, as in the inclusion of a department chair or a widely known expert in the field, another means of gaining status for the paper.

*Gift or reciprocal author:* A person included as an author solely on the basis of an understanding with another investigator that each will cite the other in order to enhance their numbers of publications, numbers usually helpful in obtaining promotions and grants.

Before investigating these strategies, we should list the criteria for authorship developed by the International Committee of Medical Journal Editors (ICMJE).[3] These include the following:

- Making a substantial contribution to the conception, or design of the study, or contributing to the analysis and interpretation of the data, or participating in data acquisition.
- Drafting the paper, or performing a critical analysis of the content.
- Finalizing approval of the paper for publication.
- Agreeing to be accountable for all aspects of the project by ensuring that questions related to the accuracy and integrity of any section of the project or paper have been investigated and resolved.

The guidelines have had a limited impact on biomedical journals, as shown by Resnik et al.,[4] who reviewed the authorship policies of 600 randomly selected journals found in the 2013

DOI: 10.1201/9781003267218-6

Thompson Reuters Journal Reports database that has 11,000 journals. Care was taken to insure representation from different fields of science. While 62.5% of the journals posted an authorship policy, 66.5% of biomedical journals had an authorship policy, statistically significantly higher than that reported from the physical sciences and engineering (54%), and mathematical sciences (50.0%). Interestingly, among the 12 policies listed by the journals, only 31.7% prohibited the use of ghost, guest, or gift authors, compared with 99% that listed criteria for authorship, in my view a significant lapse. Only 5.3% required authors to list their individual contributions. Note too that none of the journals dealt with the growing phenomenon regarding claims of equal contributions from all authors. On a positive note, the rates just described were somewhat higher than in previous studies.[4]

## Ghost and Honorary Authors

What is the extent of the problem? A widely cited study by Wislar et al.[5] examined the prevalence of honorary and ghost authors in over 800 research articles and editorial/opinion pieces in six high impact medical journals published in 2008. The journals included the *Annals of Internal Medicine, Nature Medicine, JAMA, Lancet*, the *New England Journal of Medicine*, and *PLoS Medicine*. Their approach used by Wislar et al. was simple: they surveyed the corresponding authors using a web-based questionnaire, and asked them to respond to questions regarding the use of ghost and honorary authors, with each category containing detailed definitions. (The response rate overall was 70.3%). The results were compared with those found in a 1996 study by Flanagin et al., published in 1998.[6]

Forty-nine articles (7.9%) had ghost authors, significantly fewer than the 11.5% reported in 1996, while 17.6% had honorary authorship, a non-significant change from the 19.3% reported in 1996.[6]

- *Original research reports*: Ghost authorship in 11.9%; honorary, 25%, significantly higher than the 16.3% reported in 1996
- *Reviews*: Ghost authorship in 6%, honorary, 15%
- *Editorials*: Ghost authorship in 5.3%; honorary, 11.2%

While the authors suggested that the efforts to promote responsibility and accountability had borne fruit during the years 1996–2008, the prevalence of inappropriate honorary authorship was 21% in 2008. While this was a significant decrease from the 29.2% in 1996, it still occurred in almost a quarter of the publications and was highest in original research articles. The authors also noted that the corresponding authors might have under-reported the extent of inappropriate authorship, and added that journals with lesser standards than found in these six high-impact journals might well have had higher rates. Nevertheless, when comparing 2008 with 1996, there was an overall decline in inappropriate authorship (29.1% vs 21%), no significant change in honorary authorship (19.3% vs 17.6%), and a decline in the prevalence of ghost authors (11.5% vs 7.9%).

Three years prior to the Wislar et al.[5] study, a case study by Ross et al.[7] of industry documents related to litigation over the marketing and risks of rofecoxib appeared in *JAMA*, with findings that attracted considerable attention. Some 250 court documents were analyzed, most of which focused on the internal correspondence and publication reports from Merck, along with external correspondence between Merck and medical publishing companies. All in all, 96 published articles were reviewed with regard to authorship and financial disclosure. The authors found that Merck employees, whether working independently or in collaboration with medical publishing companies, first wrote the content, and then proceeded to recruit academicians as first or second authors. The academicians were offered honoraria for their participation—although they had little or nothing to do with the research. Regarding financial disclosure, 92% of the clinical trials disclosed Merck's financial support, but only 50% of the review articles did so. In other words, the documents revealed significant evidence of ghostwriting, ghost authors, and guest authors, and led to a number of articles (cited by the authors[7]) discussing the implications for the integrity of science.

One year after the Ross et al. report,[7] Sismondo and Doucet[8] emphasized the role of publication planners whose primary role is to advance the commercialization of Pharma's research efforts. These efforts are often unacknowledged, a strategy labeled "ghost management," by the authors. Indeed, the effects of this strategy are often revealed by litigation, as in the case of rofecoxib, but also in the case of gabapentin and sertraline, to name a few. As in the rofecoxib case, Pharma recruited academics as first authors, who often failed to acknowledge the company's financial support. Pharma also hired medical educational and communication companies, with the goal of developing highly polished articles that emphasize positive results. The work of such companies is widespread, having a hand in some 40% of published clinical reports involving new products. These reports are essentially produced by a ghost management team, a strategy also stressed by Sismondo in 2007.[9]

Despite the publicity and numerous academic articles devoted to these problems, they continue. In 2015, for example, Kornhaber et al.[10] reviewed 20 research papers that focused on current issues regarding authorship. With regard to ghost authors, 21% of the surveyed authors acknowledged omitting an author, while 7.9% admitted to being ghost authors. Fifty-two percent acknowledged being listed as an honorary author at some point in their careers, with 18% suggesting coercion by the journal of academic colleagues, and 17% admitting that they had been offered an honorary authorship. In four studies cited by Kornhaber et al., the prevalence of honorary authorship ranged from 17 to 56%! The authors also noted the trend we mentioned earlier, in which more studies are claiming that all authors had contributed equally to the research—a situation not addressed by the ICMEJ.

Even more worrisome is a study by Fong and Wilhite,[11] who in 2017 published a survey of 110,000 scholars in 18 disciplines who submitted 12,000 responses. The authors found "widespread misattribution in publications and research proposals ...," to wit:

- 35.5% admitted adding authors who had contributed very little to the study. Not surprisingly, those lower in the academic hierarchy were much more likely to add a senior person. Sixty percent noted that adding a senior person would likely increase the chances of a positive review.
- 14% reported being coerced into adding a citation, with highly rated journals more likely to insist on adding a citation. (I have experienced this on occasion, but it has always come in the form of a "suggestion.")
- Females were less likely to be coerced.
- 15% admitted to adding citations of marginal significance to grant proposals, no doubt hoping to add more evidence for the proposal.

The authors concluded that the ICMJE had failed to significantly alter the problems with authorship. As we shall see in a moment, several investigators have disagreed about the extent and significance of these findings, but the flood of journals and publications would seem to call for more transparency and rigor in assessing research results. This is no small task, given data cited by Young et al.[12] showing that the number of publications in Scopus-indexed journals rose from 590,807 in 1997 to 883,853 in 2007, while 170 papers were submitted each week to *Nature,* and 12,000 were submitted to *Science.* If we look at research publications globally,[13] we find that 1,182,100 articles were published in 2003, but the numbers doubled in 2016 to 2,288,000, with China making the largest jump, from 87,000 to 426,00.

How are we to track this output? It would seem virtually impossible to ensure the integrity of each publication, but try we must. In the meantime, some have disagreed with the extent and meaning of the data just reviewed. For example, In De Tora et al.[14] reviewed the literature and found 257 papers in PubMed and 4,898 in PubMed Central. After considerable winnowing, they found 181 potentially relevant papers, of which 112 were opinion pieces. Unfortunately, there were considerable inconsistencies in definitions. Depending on the setting, definitions and methodology, the prevalence of ghostwriting ranged from less than 1% to 91%! In another systematic review,[15] Stretton also noted the varying definitions of ghostwriting and study definitions, as well as types of populations and samples, making a meta-analysis of primary estimates impossible. Stretton concluded that the evidence for prevalence of ghostwriting is "limited and can be outdated, misleading, or mistaken," harsh words indeed.

At first glance, it would appear that a valid listing of authors would be easy to achieve, but this neglects the importance placed on publications by department chairs, deans, and colleagues who sit on panels charged with promotions and awarding grants. Competition is fierce, and the drive for recognition intense, so manipulating authorship appears to be a relatively simple strategy that might enhance the odds of success.

# References

1. Cope Discussion Document (2014). What constitutes authorship? COPE Discussion Document. http://publicationethics.org/news/what-constitutes-authorship-new-cope-discussion-document. Accessed October 28, 2018.
2. McNutt, MK, et al. Transparency in authors' contributions and responsibilities to promote integrity in scientific publication. *Proceedings of the National Academy of Sciences* 2018. www.pnas.org/cgi/doi/10.1073/pnas.171574115
3. International Committee of Medical Journal Editors. Recommendations for the Conduct, Reporting, Editing, and Publication of Scholarly Work in Medical Journals 2014. http://www.icmje.org/urm_main.html
4. Resnik, DB, et al. Authorship policies of scientific journals. *Journal of Medical Ethics* 2016. https://doi.org/10.1136/medethics-2015-103171
5. Wislar, JS, et al. Honorary and ghost authorship in high impact biomedical journals: a cross sectional survey. *British Medical Journal* 2011. https://doi.org/10.1136/bmj.d6128
6. Flanagan, AA, et al. Prevalence of articles with honorary authors and ghost authors in peer-reviewed medical journals. *JAMA* 1998.
7. Ross, JS, et al. Guest authorship and ghostwriting in publications related to rofecoxib. A case study of industry documents from rofecoxib litigation. *JAMA* 2008.
8. Sismondo, S, et al. Publication ethics and the ghost management of medical publications. *Bioethics* 2010. https://doi.org/1111/j.1467-8519.01702.x
9. Sismondo, S. Ghost management: how much of the medical literature is shaped behind the scenes by the pharmaceutical industry? *Public Library of Science* 2007.
10. Kornhaber, RA, et al. Ongoing ethical issues concerning authorship in biomedical journals: an integrative review. *International Journal of Nanomedicine* 2015.
11. Fong, EA, et al. Authorship and citation manipulation in academic research. *Public Library of Science One* 2017.
12. Young, NS, et al. Why current publication practices may distort science. *Public Library of Science Medicine* 2008. https://doi.org/10.1371.journal.med.0050201,t001

13. *Science and Engineering Indicators* 2018 (NSB)-2018-1) (/statistics/2018/nsb2018/report) | Digest (NSB-2018-2) (statistics/2018/nsb2018/digest) | January 2018.
14. De Toret, LM, et al. Ghostwriting in biomedicine: a review of the published literature. *Current Medical Research and Opinion* 2019. https://doi.org/10.1080/03007995.2019.1608101
15. Streeton, S. Systematic review on the primary and secondary reporting of the prevalence of ghost-writing in the medical literature. *British Medical Journal Open* 2014. https://doi.org/10.1136/bmjopen-2013-004777

# 6

# Meta-Analyses and Systematic Reviews
## Biases and Short-Cuts to Knowledge

## Introduction

In Chapter 5, we noted that the number of scientific journals had grown to 24,000 by 2010, while the number of research publications reached 2.2 million by 2016.[1] The numbers continue to grow, but now include a remarkable increase in the numbers of predatory journals that charge exorbitant fees for publication, and offer poor or no peer review, further adding to the complexities facing meta-analyses, Indeed, concerns over these journals have led to a new field of study, Journalology,[2] a topic we shall discuss later. In any case, it seems obvious that busy clinicians, as well as investigators, have been in need of a system that would integrate and analyze the onslaught of information in order to shore up the foundation for rational prescribing. Out of this need came an emphasis on systematic reviews, followed by meta-analytic procedures applied to randomized, controlled trials. These approaches are now considered gold standards for an evidence-based approach to medicine[3,4] although concerns are mounting with regard to bias.[4]

## Basics

Before getting to contemporary concerns, let's examine the history of these developments, as described by de Vrieze in his essay on the meta-wars in 2018.[5] He noted that Gene Glass, a statistician at the University of Colorado, had coined the term meta-analysis in 1976. Glass also introduced the concept of a systematic review, whereby the investigator develops a set of pre-defined search and selection criteria that are used in examining the literature on a topic of interest. Studies that do not meet the predefined criteria are excluded. Should the review yield fairly similar quantitative data, a meta-analysis can be conducted. There is no doubt about the popularity of meta-analyses, with the numbers growing from less than 1,000 in the year 2000 to about 11,000 in 2017.[5] (We now have meta-analyses of meta-analyses!) Oddly enough, despite the popularity and pervasiveness of systematic reviews and meta-analyses, neither term can be found in the index of *The American Psychiatric Association Publishing Textbook of Psychiatry*,[6, pp.1263–1326] published in 2019, thus missing an opportunity for the early education of psychiatry trainees, not to speak of faculty.

The basics of a meta-analysis include applying a variety of statistical tests to the results of a systematic review, such that the results of individual studies can be combined and reported in several ways, including an effect size (ES). This is a measure of the difference between, say,

DOI: 10.1201/9781003267218-7

the efficacy of a medication vs another treatment, and is more informative than simply using a *p* value of 0.05. After all, the *p* value is an arbitrary number that denotes statistical significance, but does not give the clinician any idea of the magnitude or precision of the treatment,[7,8] values important to rational prescribing. These can be obtained by calculating the standardized ES, Cohen's D, which uses an actual number, say a percentage, divided the standard deviation, a measure of variability. The ES can be further defined by a confidence interval (CI), which gives us a range of plausible values for the ES, and the likelihood that the reported ES would be captured in 95% of trials. A small ES is about 0.2, and a medium or moderate ES is about 0.5, capturing a treatment result thought to be obvious to the naked eye.[7] However, there is not universal agreement on these definitions, with Ghaemi[8] stating that an ES or 0.4 or smaller is low, 0.4–0.7 is medium, and above 0.7 is large.

## Odds ratios and relative risks

When the outcome is couched in terms of a dichotomous variable, a research question that can be answered yes or no (how many patients relapsed or died after an event?), one can use an odds ratio (OR). The odds ratio is simply a measure of the association between an event and an outcome, divided by the association between those not exposed to the event and an outcome. Let's say we are investigating the number of people who became ill after eating ice cream (13/17) vs the number who did not become ill (32/23). We divide the two results (13/17) divide by 32/33 and find an OR of 0.55. Another term is relative risk (RR), wherein the number of patients who relapsed or died is divided by the total number of patients in the study. Note that statisticians state that the OR can be similar to the RR. This can occur when the incidence of the disease is less than 10%. If higher than 10%, the OR will exaggerate the RR. One can further assess the results of studies via two models, one being a fixed effects model. This model assumes that among all of the groups being studied, there is a true mean ES. The other is a random effects model, a model which assumes that each study can have a true mean ES that differs from the others, perhaps due to study conditions.

# General Problems with the Meta-Analytic Approach

Despite the advances in combing and analyzing multiple studies that collectively have hundreds of subjects, problems remain. On a general level, Ghaemi[8] has stressed the inherent difficulties in combing disparate studies into a pool, since the studies themselves are often quite heterogeneous. However, virtually all well-done meta-analyses control for heterogeneity. Ghaemi further notes that the "statistical alchemy" of meta-analyses might discourage further study of the issues at hand, but investigators often take a dim view of previous studies, whether meta-analytic or not. Indeed, investigators are often more than eager to top whatever the older studies discovered—a process that is part of the rhetoric of science, and a potential path to fame and fortune, or, at the very least, promotion. Ghaemi further observes that a methodologically sound single study can yield results more informative than a meta-analysis. The problem here is that many studies in psychiatry and the social sciences are not sufficiently well-powered. This is particularly true of imaging research,[9] which has dominated biological studies in mental health. Indeed, small sample size was a prominent issue in a scathing critique by Ioannidis in 2016 of meta-analyses and systematic reviews.[10] Indeed, he noted that only 3% of recent meta-analytic studies had been adequately conducted, such that they could provide clinicians with useful information.

# Specific Issues

## Bias

Starting with a systematic review, there are numerous steps that can lead to bias in the ultimate outcomes.[5] The reader may recall that investigators start with a specific question and develop detailed sets of inclusion and exclusion criteria that set the pace for acceptance of studies. These can include specific time periods during which the relevant studies have been accomplished, in which case entire classes of drugs or other treatments may have been excluded. Only peer-reviewed published studies are accepted, in which case a large literature involving unpublished studies are excluded, many of which have negative results, as we have seen previously. Limits are usually set on the length of the investigation, thus neglecting serious questions regarding the long-term outcome of treatments, a question of great interest to patients, families, and clinicians. Other problems include bias in the selection criteria resulting from adjusting the criteria to ensure the inclusion[5] of articles well-known to investigators already aware of the most significant, high-impact papers, raising the possibility of bias, whether overt or unwittingly.

Even Cochrane Reviews (CRs), usually held to be a gold standard for evidence-based medicine, have had problems. For example, Deshpande et al.,[11] examined the risk of bias across a variety of topics studied in 3,836 non-Cochrane Reviews and 568 CRs published from 2010 onward. The good news: 87% of the CRs were at low risk of bias, compared with only 12% of non-Cochrane Reviews. The bad news: the total number of non-Cochrane Reviews was far higher, at 17,67 vs 1,153 CRs, which of course means that the literature may be dominated by systematic reviews at high risk of bias! The authors cautioned that even CRs may be biased, but in far smaller numbers. The divide between CRs and non-CR systematic reviews was emphasized by another study of outcomes,[12] with non-CRs being twice as likely to yield positive conclusions. In another study,[13] a randomly selected sample of published systematic reviews and meta-analyses was compared with 36 completed reviews found in the Cochrane Database of Systematic Reviews. The goal: to examine any methodological differences in results reported in the two groups. While there were no differences in trial sources, descriptions of effect estimates, or testing for heterogeneity, CRs more often assessed quality of the trials, and provided detailed descriptions of the inclusion and exclusion criteria. Two years after the study was completed, the authors noted that half of the CRs had been updated, but only one of the non-CR reviews.

Another threat to the validity of systematic reviews and meta-analyses rests on the presence of biases within the studies selected for inclusion, a problem we've addressed in previous chapters. However, we should note an additional examination[14] of a series of 16 cohort studies that assessed publication and outcome reporting biases in RCTs. Three of these studies found that studies with statistically significant outcomes were twice to four times as likely to be published vs those with non-significant outcomes, similar to results we've reviewed previously. Making matters worse, 40–62% of studies had at least one primary outcome that was introduced, omitted, or changed! Sadly, these practices may well undercut the results of systematic reviews and meta-analytic studies.

## Industry and non-industry funding of meta-analytic studies: Does this bias the outcome?

Unfortunately, this appears to be the case. Twelve years ago, Jørgensen et al.[4] investigated 39 meta-analyses that compared different drugs or classes of drugs, and divided them into those with industry support, non-profit support, no support, and undeclared support. The authors used a validated scale (0–7) to judge the methodological quality. Industry-supported meta-analyses ranked considerably lower on quality, with a median score of 2.5, vs 6 for non-industry supported studies, a significant difference. Significant differences were found in non-industry vs industry supported studies with non-industry supported studies having fewer faults in the avoidance of selection bias, better reporting of allocation concealment and assessing validity of the selected studies, and reporting of procedures aimed at blinding. About 40% of industry-sponsored meta-analyses recommended the experimental drug without reservations, compared with 22% of meta-analyses funded by a non-profit, or without funding.

A Cochrane Review[15] in 2013 also found that industry-sponsored studies resulted in a 24% increase in positive results, less harm, and more favorable conclusions when compared with non-industry sponsored studies. However, there were no methodological differences in the two approaches, leaving the possibility of selective reporting, dosing, and choice of comparators as important factors. In an updated Cochrane Review published in 2017,[16] the authors added 27 new papers investigating the results of industry-sponsorship of drugs and devices, and again noted that industry-sponsorship was associated with a 27% increase in favorable results and a 34% increase in favorable conclusions. However, industry sponsorship did have a lower risk of bias with regard to blinding.

Another source of difficulties lies in the failure of some studies to document any conflicts of interest (COIs) in studies selected for a meta-analysis. This was noted by Roseman et al.[17] who found that none of the 29 meta-analyses of pharmacological treatments investigated the possibility of COIs in the selected studies. In another meta-analysis[18] of pharmacotherapy vs psychotherapy in adult depression, there were five instances where authors of the original investigations had failed to report on existing COIs. However, this failed to have any significant effect on the primary finding of a subtle but consistently small effect favoring pharmacotherapy. In a review of 106 systematic reviews, Brugha et al.[19] in 2012 emphasized that many reviews failed to describe study quality, publication bias, confounding, and the methods used for data extraction. Studies are further complicated by the use of widely varying instruments used to measure the results of treatment. Some rating scales, for instance, are novel, and have not been validated.

We have focused on pharmacological studies, but a review[20] of industry funding in controlled trials (n=110) of devices, implants, drugs, and surgical techniques, also found a highly significant effect of industry sponsorship. While the overall quality of the studies (primarily involving drugs) was good, 78% of the studies sponsored by industry published a favorable conclusion, with a remarkably high odds ratio of 23.35! Interestingly, 85% of the studies had been published in one journal, the *Journal of Neurosurgery*.

# Conclusions

Another problem for clinicians: the existence of overlapping meta-analysis and separate meta-analyses on the same topic. Given the problems just noted, it may not be surprising to learn that meta-analyses of the same subject have reached contradictory conclusions,[5] as in the case of placebo responses to antidepressants, while overlapping meta-analyses of the same issue have also been contradictory.[21] It is clear that readers of meta-analyses must cast a skeptical eye on the results, and look for COI, consistency of results across studies, and acknowledgment of potential biases in the original investigations. Let's now proceed to another issue: the reproducibility of research results, and whether the results are stable over time.

# References

1. Larsen, PI, et al. The rate of growth in scientific publication and decline in coverage provided by Science Citation Index. *Scientometrics* 2010.
2. Couzin-Frankel, J. Journals under the microscope. *Science* 2018.
3. Harbour, RR, et al. A new system for grading recommendations in evidence-based guidelines. *British Medical Journal* 2001.
4. Jørgensen, AW, et al. Industry-supported meta-analyses compared with meta-analyses with non-profit or no support: differences in methodological quality and conclusions. *BMC Medical Research Methodology* 2008. https://doi.org/10.1186/1471-2288-8-60
5. de Vrieze, J. The metawars. Meta-analyses were supposed to end scientific debates. Often, they only cause more controversy. *Science* 2018.
6. *The American Psychiatric Association Publishing Textbook of Psychiatry*, 7th Edition. Editor: Roberts, LW, 2019.
7. Cohen, J. *Statistical Power Analysis for the Behavioral Sciences*, Revised Edition. Academic Press, New York, 1977.
8. Ghaemi, SN. The alchemy of meta-analysis. In, *A Clinician's Guide to Statistics and Epidemiology in Mental Health*. New York, Cambridge University Press, 2009.
9. Button, KS, et al. Power failure: why small sample size undermines the reliability of neuroscience. *Nature Reviews|Neuroscience* 2013.
10. Ioannidis, JPA. The mass production of redundant, misleading, and conflicted systematic reviews and meta-analyses. *Milbank Quarterly* 2016.
11. Deshpande, S, et al. Not all Cochrane Reviews are good quality systematic reviews. *Value in Health* 2016. Meeting abstract PRM77.
12. Tricco, AC, et al. Non-Cochrane Reviews were twice as likely to have positive conclusion statements; cross-sectional study. *Journal of Clinical Epidemiology* 2009.
13. Jadad, AR, et al. Methodology and reports of systematic reviews and meta-analyses. A comparison of Cochrane Reviews with articles published in paper-based journals. *JAMA* 1998.
14. Dwan, K, et al. Systematic review of the empirical evidence of study publication bias and outcome reporting bias. *Public Library of Science One* 2008. https://doi.org/10.1371/journalpone.003081
15. Bero, L. Industry sponsorship and research outcome. A Cochrane Review. *JAMA Internal Medicine* 2013.
16. Lundh, A, et al. Industry sponsorship and research outcome. *Cochrane Database Systematic Reviews* 2017. https://doi.org/0.1002/14651858.MR000033.put
17. Roseman, J, et al. Reporting on conflicts of interest in meta-analyses of trials of pharmacological treatments. *JAMA* 2011:305:1008–1017
18. Cristea, IA, et al. Sponsorship bias in the comparative efficacy of psychotherapy and pharmacotherapy for adult depression: meta-analysis. *British Journal of Psychiatry* 2017. https://doi.org/10.1192/bjp.bp.115.179275
19. Brugha, TS, et al. Methodology and reporting of systematic reviews and meta-analyses of observational studies in psychiatric epidemiology: systematic review. *British Journal of Psychiatry* 2018. https://doi.org/10.1192/bjp.bp.111.098103
20. Khan, NR, et al. A review of industry funding in randomized controlled trials published in the neurosurgical literature-the elephant in the room [review]. *Neurosurgery* 2018:83:890–897
21. Siontis, KC, et al. Overlapping meta-analyses on the same topic: survey of published studies. *British Medical Journal* 2013. 347f14501. https://doi.org/10.1136/bmj.f4501

# 7

# Replication and Reproducibility of Research Results
## A Crisis?

## Introduction

Replication and reproducibility of scientific studies have been topics of interest for decades, with the emphasis on validation of research findings dating to Robert Boyle's insistence in the 17th century that an experiment must be witnessed in order to ensure its veracity.[1] During this century, interest in validation has grown substantially, but not in the fashion that Boyle recommended, given the flood of journals and publications, a development that makes hiring independent observers impractical, not only financially, but secondary to privacy regulations.[2] Indeed, a visit to the Web of Science database in September 2020,[3] found 1,644 citations published over the past 5 years that focused on reproducibility and replication. Some authors have said that problems in these areas are indicative of a crisis for science.[4,5] In 2017, Ionannidis[6] emphasized that problems in validation are not isolated to clinical research, but are also found in basic and preclinical research—including an area of immense clinical interest, cancer biology.

## First: Problems with definitions

Before honing in on specific fields of interest, we must acknowledge inconsistencies in the definitions of reproducibility and replicability.[2,7,8] According to Guttenger,[2] replication is an attempt at reproducing an earlier experiment or finding, while replicability refers to the quality of an experiment or observation. In addition, some suggest that we separate direct replication from conceptual replications. A direct replication uses the same experimental protocol and the same experimental materials, such as a set of antibodies or a specific population. The outcome should be similar, either exactly so, or at least in the same direction, but the limits are not well-defined. By way of contrast, a conceptual replication involves an attempt to achieve an outcome similar to that of the original experiment, but uses a different protocol and/or materials.[2]

However, Goodman et al.,[7] cites a subcommittee report from the National Science Foundation[8] in which reproducibility refers to a process in which an investigator duplicates the results of a previous study by using the same materials, analysis files, and statistical analyses in an attempt to obtain the same results. This seems equivalent to the concept of a direct replication as just defined. The National Science Foundation added that the ability to reproduce a study is a minimum necessary condition for a finding to be both believable and informative."[8] Goodman et al.[7] also note that the definitions reproducibility and replication are sometimes reversed. Unfortunately, these definitions have not provided clear operational criteria that

DOI: 10.1201/9781003267218-8

would define standards of success. Goodman et al. therefore proposed a new terminology with descriptors for the underlying construct of reproducibility, including:

- *Methods reproducibility*: Using the same experimental conditions and computational tools.
- *Results reproducibility*: Using the same experimental methods in a new study in order to corroborate the previous results.
- *Inferential reproducibility*: Where the investigator claims equivalent knowledge from a replication or a new analysis.

Whether this approach will bear fruit is not clear, but has been recommended by others.[1] However, what we need to emphasize is simple: Are the research results are valid?[7, p.1]

## What is the extent of the problem?

In 2016, Baker[5] published a summary of the results obtained from a survey of 1,576 investigators who responded to a questionnaire on reproducibility in research. Fifty-two percent agreed that there was a significant crisis in reproducibility, but less than a third thought that the failure to reproduce meant that the initial results were wrong. Indeed, most said they trusted the literature, despite labeling the problem a crisis! Yet 41% of those working in internal medicine noted that their labs had undertaken steps to enhance reproducibility, and 90% endorsed a series of steps aimed at improving reproducibility. Seventy percent admitted that they had tried but failed to reproduce the results of another investigator's research. Over half had failed to reproduce their own experiments, and more than 20% noted that they had been contacted by other researchers who had been unable to reproduce their own work. On the other hand, 24% said they had published a successful replication, while 13% had published a failed replication. Only 12% indicated that they had been unable to publish any successful replications. Remarkably, 73% said they could trust at least half of the papers in their field, but how can this indicate confidence, when there is a 50% chance that a given paper cannot be trusted?

## Basic and preclinical research: Problems and solutions

Another paper[9] in 2015 attracted a good deal of attention when the authors reported that 75–90% of published studies are not reproducible. One consequence: a waste of $29 billion yearly on unsuccessful efforts at reproducing preclinical research.[10] As I mentioned earlier, concerns have been raised in recent years with regard to reproducibility in basic and preclinical research, with Ioannidis[6] noting that publications from leading academic medical centers have found reproducibility rates of only 11% to 25%—including studies of cancer biology (more on this below). Why are rates so low? Ioannidis stresses the complex biology of humans, but notes as well incomplete reporting of subtle changes in cell cultures and experimental manipulations in animals that can affect outcome. When compared with clinical research, preclinical research is notable for:

- Smaller sample sizes
- Limited familiarity with statistical methods
- Lack of randomization
- Poor or absent blinding
- Poor methods of randomization

Ioannidis also states that peer reviews of complex studies are unavoidably superficial, a problem that might be helped by pre-registration and more transparency.[6] In a separate paper, Begley and Ioannidis[9] also recommend that institutions require their investigators to not only retain raw data, but submit it to other investigators on request. Obviously, many investigators might respond by claiming that such data belongs to the pharmaceutical company or university, and might contain trade secrets. The debate continues.

In support of the above critique, Miyakawa, the editor of *Molecular Brain* in 2020, summarized the results of an examination of 180 manuscripts received from 2017 and later.[4] He noted that he had sent 41 of these for revision, principally due to the lack of raw data, so asked for the raw data, including images using Western blotting, size markers, quantified numerical data for each sample, absolute $p$-values, and corrections for multiple tests where necessary. Remarkably, 21 of the 41 papers were withdrawn without sending the raw data, while the editor rejected 19 of the remaining 20 because the submitted data were incomplete. Miyakawa suggested that, at least in part, the raw data may not have existed, but noted that the National Institute of Mental Health now requires that all NIMH-funded investigators deposit all raw and analyzed data into its informatic infrastructure. Should journals make the same requirement? In principle, this is appealing, but would it be financially viable?[10]

Other studies have sounded the alarm over in vivo research. For example, Reichlin et al.[11] surveyed all registered in vivo investigators in Switzerland, but only 16% returned completed questionnaire asking about the use and reporting of measures aimed at minimizing bias. A critical issue: their use of ARRIVE Guidelines, a set of 20 recommendations for ensuring proper animal research. The use of these guidelines had been endorsed by over 1,000 journals. Over 60% of respondents indicated they were knowledgeable about the risks of bias stemming from selective reporting, selection bias, and detection bias, and had avoided such risks in their own research. While at least half were aware of publication bias, only 15–41% were concerned about these biases in their own research! With regard to the ARRIVE Guidelines,[12] 56% said they had never heard of them! Reichlin et al. also stressed[11] that the self-reports of respondents with regard to measures they had taken against biases were considerably higher than reports found in systematic reviews of the literature, indicating that they might be overestimating their own performance. The results of this survey prompted the authors to recommend increased educational efforts with regard to scientific integrity in animal experiments, but questioned the use of self-reports as a reliable measure of the validity of such efforts.

Similar concerns have been raised about the integrity of in vitro research, where high standards of reproducibility and reliability should be established in order to minimize error.[13] For clinicians, the question of flawed animal and in vitro research may seem somewhat less important to the prescribing process, but this work is the foundation on which the development, efficacy, and safety of drugs and devices rests. It cannot be ignored or minimized.

## Clinical studies in reproducibility: Traumatic brain injury and brain asymmetry

Given the growing importance of detecting and managing traumatic brain injury (TBI), there is agreement that the use of functional brain imaging (fMRI; BOLD fMRI) holds considerable promise in advancing the care of those so afflicted. However, Olsen et al.[14] have noted that the heterogeneity of the population, combined with small sample sizes in many studies, have resulted in significant barriers to scientific progress and clinical usefulness. In a lengthy review of these issues, Poldrack et al.[15] focused first on statistical power, noting that sample sizes have increased over the past 20 years, with sizes greater than 100 found in only 8 studies in 2012 but in 17 studies in 2015. Nevertheless, the median group size in 2014 for fMRI studies with multiple groups was only 19 subjects, considerably lower than the recommendation for a minimum of 20 subjects per cell.

Clearly, a sample size of 19 would be likely to detect only relatively large effect sizes. The authors also noted insufficient reporting of data analysis and parameters, with the choice of analyses based, at least in part, on the observed data! Obviously, this can inflate Type I error rates, but this kind of manipulation could be avoided by prespecifying the methodology. Other problems include a lack of correction for multiple tests, or combining different approaches and thresholds that lead to many undocumented researcher degrees of freedom.[15, p.8] Yet more problems stem from errors in custom-made software programs designed for individual projects, flaws in study reports, and the lack of quantitative evidence and/or the lack of appropriate tests for statistical interactions.

Unfortunately, the authors[15] found very few examples of direct replication in neuroimaging. They cited one attempt at replicating 17 studies that had found an association between brain structure and behavior, but only one of the attempts found evidence of an effect size as equivalent to that found in the original study. In addition, 8 of the 17 replication studies found stronger evidence for a null effect. At the end of the paper, the authors demonstrated evidence showing that even a set of random data can yield a correlation between brain and behavior, if one uses uncorrected statistics and circular regions of interest analyses.

The power of larger sample sizes is nicely illustrated by a study[16] on brain-asymmetry research that used summary statistics from the ENIGMA cortical asymmetry project,[17] an investigation that had used data from 17,441 healthy subjects from 99 separate MRI datasets gathered from around the world. This project had aimed to map left-right asymmetries in regional measurements of surface areas and cortical thickness. The present study[16] examined hemispheric asymmetries with regard to reproducibility. Reproducibility was defined as present when the effect within a database matched the meta-analytic effect from 98 other data sets, in terms of the significance threshold and direction of the effect. The authors found an average reproducibility rate of 63.2% (SD = 22.9%, min = 22.2%, max = 97.0%), but noted that these findings took place in an excellent publishing environment, with no selective reporting or $p$ hacking. In this case, and contrary to the concerns noted earlier, heterogeneity was of limited significance. The authors also stressed that in the original project,[17] MRI quality control, processing, and analyses were harmonized, thus eliminating the problems encountered when different strategies are used in studies involving MRI, as noted earlier by Poldrack et al.[15]

The conclusion: It appears that size of the dataset and the true effect size were the primary drivers of reproducibility, rather than subject age, scanner field strength, regional size, the software version, or the reliability of cortical regional measurements. Yet these factors have continued to play significant roles in neuroimaging generally, as noted above. Given the diversity of strategies, scanners, and statistical methods used in centers across the United States, it's difficult to imagine that harmonization can be achieved, leaving clinicians still grasping to reconcile the diverse results. Indeed, in neuroscience, the median statistical power of studies is estimated to be 21%, indicating that of 100 studies (assuming that the principal finding is true and accurately estimated), only 21 would detect statistically significant evidence supporting the finding.[18] However, this stands in marked contrast to a positive result rate of 85% in neuroscience generally,[19] a result rate so high that it indicates suppression of negative results and inflation of positive results.

## Cancer biology and reproducibility

Concerns over reproducibility in cancer biology research appear to be justified. Indeed, the lack of reproducibility may hinder discoveries of new drugs that could positively affect the treatment of cancer and other illnesses. In one effort to clarify the frequency and causes of this problem, Mobley et al.[20] surveyed the staff and trainees at the MD Anderson Cancer Center using a 20-item anonymous online questionnaire asking about their experiences in reproducing findings from published studies. The overall response rate was only 14.75%, even less than in the Reichlin et al. study[11] noted earlier! Of the respondents, 54% said they had tried to reproduce a finding, but had not been able to do so. In addition, authors of the non-reproducible papers had been contacted for further information and clarification, but 18% did not reply, and 43% responded with indifference or negativity. We should note too that one-third of trainees reported that they were pressured to prove their mentors' hypotheses, even though their own data did not support it.

Given the high rate of non-response to the survey, one suspects that the results might have been even more damaging, but, coming from a prestigious cancer center, the data are still worrisome. The authors claimed that academic expectations at all levels appeared to be the principal driver of their findings, but this is an observation not supported by others,[21] as we shall discuss. Nevertheless, other studies have confirmed failures in reproducibility in cancer research, including a report by Begley and Ellis,[22] who noted that attempts at replicating 53 preclinical studies at Amgen biotechnology succeeded in only 6%, while at Bayer Health Care, only 25% of published preclinical studies could be validated to the point where the projects could continue.[23]

## What to do?

In response to these findings, Errington et al.[24] launched the Reproducibility Project: Cancer Biology, in which they plan to replicate 50 high-impact cancer biology studies published in 2010–2012. The plan involves replicating a subset of experimental results from each study, after first developing detailed experimental designs for the replications and subjecting them to peer review before publication. The final results will be described in a Replication Study. However, the Project has been downsized to 29 papers, in part secondary to budget limitations, Baker and Dolgin[25] also report that 5 of the first 7 studies have yielded a murky picture. This seems especially true of one study, but I will omit the details, given the ongoing debate. The authors noted, however, that the five muddy studies are being published by another journal and list the citations. These citations were also acknowledged in a 2017 viewpoint by Nosek and Errington,[26] who outlined the difficulties faced by the Project, including misjudging the importance of certain methodologies, mistaking noise for signals, and neglecting the importance of contamination of cell lines.

More generally, the authors[25] also stressed the lack of a straightforward answer as to what counts as a successful replication. Despite a rigorous approach to the project, reproducibility in cancer biology is considerably more difficult than expected. Are there similar problems in the social sciences, including psychology?

## Social sciences and replication, reproducibility

Before discussing reproducibility in psychology, let's first discuss the results of an investigation[27] into transparency and reproducibility in the social sciences generally, including economics, econometrics and finance, psychology, business, management, and accounting.

A random sampling of the literature in 2014–2017 yielded 250 articles from a database of over 485,000. Despite the emphasis on transparency in recent years, only 40% of the articles were publicly available, and 54% were available only via a paywall, although at least 25% had received public funding. Six percent could not be retrieved by any method! None contained a protocol or materials availability statement. No articles had been pre-registered. Sixty-nine percent did not include a statement on funding, while 85% did not report COIs. Only 1% of the articles self-identified as a replication study, while 11% were included in an evidence synthesis in a meta-analysis. Articles containing detailed empirical data were rarely cited.

The authors concluded the obvious: that the social sciences have been lacking in transparency and reproducibility, despite the potential costs to the integrity and efficiency of science, not to speak of the effects on clinicians. However, another group undertook a replication[28] of experimental studies in social sciences published in *Science and Nature* between 2010 and 2015, where the results were more encouraging. Indeed, 62% of studies found a signal in the same direction as noted in the original studies, *but* the effect size was about 50% of the original effect size. Additional analyses indicated that false positives and inflated effect sizes strongly contributed to the problems with reproducibility, as shown too by Simmons et al.[29]

## Replication in psychology

In 2012, Makel et al.[30] cited several studies showing that replications of investigations in psychological sciences had been met in the literature with disparaging comments about their originality and prestige. However, the authors stressed that there had been no systematic studies of the prevalence of such studies, so they undertook a review of replications in psychological sciences published since 1900 in 100 psychology journals with the highest 5-year impact factors. They used the search term "replicat," to identify relevant articles, and then calculated the frequency of replications in each journal. In addition, they randomly selected 500 articles containing the term "replicat," in order to assess whether an article was a new replication, and whether it was considered a success or failure. What were the results?

The term "replicat" was used in only 1.57% of the journals with a range of 0%–6%. Reflecting the growing interest in replication, usage of the term after the year 2000 increased by 84% over the period from 1950 to 1999. Nevertheless, the overall replication rate was only 1.07%, but a majority of these were considered successful. In 2020,[31] a meta-review of the meta-analytic studies in psychology also noted that over three decades, emphasis on transparent reporting had increased significantly. Unfortunately, studies often failed to report specific search results, data extraction procedures, effect sizes, and moderators. The omission of such factors clearly constitute a barrier to reproducibility.

Perhaps the most well-known study of replication/reproducibility was the Open Science Collaboration,[32] wherein the authors developed a detailed protocol for conducting well-powered and high-powered replications of 100 studies, yielding an open data set. They developed 5 indicators of replication, including:

- Evaluation of the replication effect against the null hypothesis of no effect, using $p > .05$ to test whether the replication was in the same direction of the original study. Remarkably, 97% of the original studies had positive effects, but this fell to 36.1% in the replications.
- Evaluation of the replication effect against the original effect size. In this evaluation, one tests whether the original effect size falls within the 95% confidence interval of the effect size estimate from the replication. Overall, the data suggested a 47.4% replication success rate.

- Comparison of the original and replication effect sizes. Overall, the magnitude of the original effect sizes was larger than the replication effect sizes. This was the case in 82.8% of the original studies.
- Combing the original and replication effect sizes for cumulative evidence. This produced a 70% rate of significant results, but his assumed no publication bias in the original results, a questionable assumption, given the frequency of publication bias.
- A subjective assessment of "did it replicate?" Thirty-eight percent of the replications were subjectively rated as successful.

In summary, successful replication seemed most consistently related to the original strength of the evidence, including the original *p-value* and the effect size, rather than the expertise of the original or replication teams, and how the replication was done. However, the author concluded that a large portion of the replications did not reproduce the evidence supporting the original results, despite careful planning of the replication strategies. On the other hand, the authors cautioned us that science progresses by a combination of verification of prior results and innovation. Indeed, first results are seldom consistently valid, and are subject to correction and/or invalidation.

Not surprisingly, the Open Science Collaboration study[32] generated considerable criticism, including an article by Gilbert et al.,[33] who noted several statistical errors that not only invalidated the conclusion, but showed that reproducibility was quite high. In a detailed response, Anderson et al.,[34] of the Open Science Collaboration, pointed out that the Gilbert et al. study[33] was limited by statistical misconceptions and their use of selectively interpreted correlational data. Anderson et al. stated that both optimistic and pessimistic conclusions are possible, but neither is warranted! Another point of view was raised in 2019, wherein Bressan[35] noted that replications may themselves be as unreliable as the original studies, in part secondary to the failure to treat the new data any differently from the old. This alleged failure appears to be based on the reluctance to use post-hoc strategies that might discover unexpected confounds and biases. Bressan then proceeded to illustrate her point by noting several such confounds in a number of failed replications in the Open Science study, including one of her own.

Beyond the debate over methodology, statistics, and other technical issues, others have accused replication investigators of, bullying, lacking originality, and fostering a culture of shaming.[36,37] Given the obvious threats to one's reputation and integrity, I can understand the concerns, but, as noted earlier, replications have long been thought to be crucial to scientific integrity, and should be continued.

## Replication, reproducibility in psychiatry

A search[38] of the Web of Science on October 10, 2020 revealed only 42 hits under the search term "reproducibility and psychiatry," much in contrast to psychology and cancer. This was noted as well in a 2020 systematic review[39] of transparency and reproducibility in 296 articles published in psychiatry journals over a 5-year period. Only 17 articles provided access to the data necessary for a study of reproducibility, with only 4 posted an in-depth protocol. One hundred and seven were available online, but very few described the study hypotheses, methods, and analyses. While the authors admit that the sample size was small, the data clearly indicates significant barriers to the reproducibility of psychiatric research.

Indeed, the term "replication" was used in a study[40] of highly cited research papers in psychiatry that were tracked a decade after publication in order to gauge how the original findings held up. The authors selected 3 general medicine and 5 psychiatry journals with the highest impact factors in the year 2000, and then selected 83 studies that had found effective treatments. Each study had been cited at least 30 times in the 3 years following publication. Only 16 had been replicated, but, in this paper, the term replication was used very loosely. In fact, subsequent investigators had simply addressed the primary clinical question, but had not attempted to reproduce the methodology. Instead, the follow-up studies often had a better design, or similar designs with a larger sample. In any case, another 16 studies were contradicted, and 11 were found to have substantially smaller effect sizes, with the standardized mean differences of the initial studies overestimated by 132%!

A lesson for clinicians: even studies published in high-impact, major journals with high citation rates, may not hold up over time. This is especially true if the sample size was small, and the effect size large. But sample size in psychiatry is not the only significant problem with regard to studies of reproducibility; marked heterogeneity is another. For example, using DSM-5 criteria for the diagnosis of major depressive disorder, there are 227 different symptom pictures, a number that increases to 10,377 if one uses the qualitative differences, and up to 341,737 unique profiles if one adds the criteria for melancholia.[41] In the STAR*D studies of major depressive disorder, Fried and Nesse[42] found 1,030 symptom profiles. In schizophrenia, heterogeneity is present in the course, response to medications, age of onset, symptoms, genetics, and environmental risk factors.[43] Unfortunately, another major problem is the lack of a diagnostically useful biomarker for any mental disorder.[44]

Yet Kochunov et al.,[43] while emphasizing heterogeneity in schizophrenia, point with optimism to a recent study by Alnæs et al.[45] who compared variability in brain structure in subjects with schizophrenia ($n$ = 1,151) and healthy controls ($n$ = 2,010). They asked whether such variability is associated with the polygenic risk score (PRS). However, Alnæs et al., quantified sources of patient-control differences in individual deviations from the mean, rather than the traditional approach used in meta-analyses, where published mean effect sizes are used in group-level comparisons. Patients had higher heterogeneity in measurements of brain structures than did controls, but the effect sizes of the patient-control differences were much smaller than the effect size of the group difference. Indeed, brain structural heterogeneity goes beyond the mean differences, and may reflect higher sensitivity to environmental and genetic perturbations that are not captured by the PRS.

However, Kochunov et al., in their editorial[43] on the results of this study, noted that this approach might provide a new method of not only examining individual heterogeneity, but reproducibility of studies on schizophrenia. Yet the authors also noted the small effect sizes in the PRS data compared with the mean effect size, and questioned whether this approach could be reproducible On the other hand, they noted that the methodology was similar to that found in several prior studies of neuroimaging using big data, so plotted the t scores of the patient-control differences in Alnæs et al.,[45] vs the effect sizes in the previously published work. This approach found a "remarkable correlation" of coefficients of 0.98, giving hope that imaging studies that aggregate big data might yield high rates of reproducibility.

We should note that the combination of effect sizes, very large sample sizes, and independent replication across multiple samples fulfills the recommendations found in a recent editorial[46] on leveraging statistical methods to improve validity and reproducibility of research. Similarly, a study[47] of the reproducibility of white matter microstructural measures in data collected 1 year apart in youths of families with and without a history of substance use disorders, found excellent reproducibility of fractional anisotropy values. Interestingly, there was no significant effect of family history on reproducibility. Unfortunately, earlier studies in imaging sometimes failed to enroll adequate samples, as we have stressed.[6,18] For example, in a study of fMRI activation during a story listening task in 10 patients with schizophrenia and 10 healthy controls, fMRI sessions 21 months apart found a high degree of overlap in the activation maps, but the sample size clearly limits the results.[48]

In marked contrast, the Cognitive Genetics Collaboration (COCORO)[49] has successfully replicated studies by the Enigma Collaboration (Enhancing Neuroimaging Genetics through Meta-analysis) in schizophrenia, including volumetric changes, white matter microstructural alterations, and subcortical regional volume changes. The COCORO study also found similar white matter alterations in bipolar disorder, schizophrenia, and autism spectrum disorder. but not in major depression. Sample sizes ranged from 126 to 2,359. This is very impressive work, despite the problems associated with big data.[50]

In summary, the reproducibility of research in mental health can be improved[51] by implementing the following:

- Pre-registration of hypotheses and analyses
- Putting the materials used online
- Publishing the analysis codes
- Making the data openly available
- Making use of pre-prints
- Shifting of organizational priorities such that more value is given to sound scientific methods and questions, regardless of results
- Emphasizing the value of transparency and reproducibility early in training

Finally, despite the many editorials, essays, and articles on reproducibility, Fanelli[52] has marshaled evidence showing that the argument for a crisis in reproducibility is somewhat misguided, particularly with regard to the idea that the crisis has engulfed entire disciplines. Indeed, evidence suggests that subfields in any given area are more likely to be associated with flawed research, especially in those investigations with low power and low levels of potential reproducibility. Nevertheless, she notes studies indicating that problems such as $p$-hacking are not severely distorting the general literature. In addition, she cites studies showing higher levels of reproducibility than those cited earlier in this paper, and insists that the problem has not worsened over time. We shall take up that issue later. Let's now move to an examination of the problems associated with reporting of outcomes.

# References

1. Mullane, K, Williams, M. Enhancing reproducibility: failures from reproducibility initiatives underline core challenges. *Biochemical Pharmacology* 2017. http://dx.doi.org/10.1016/j.bcp.2017.04.008
2. Guttinger, S. The limits of replicability. *European Journal of Philosophy of Science* 2020. https://doi.org.1007/s13194-019-0269-1
3. Web of Science database, accessed September 22, 2020.
4. Miyakawa, T. No raw data, no science: another possible source of the reproducibility crisis *Molecular Brain* 2020. https://doi.org/10.1186/s13041-020-0552-2
5. Baker, M. Is there a reproducibility crisis? *Nature* 2016.
6. Ioannidis, JPA. Acknowledging and overcoming nonreproducibility in basic and preclinical research. *JAMA* 2017. https://doi.org/10.1001/jama.2017.0549
7. Goodman, SN, et al. What does research reproducibility mean? *Science Translational Medicine* 2016.
8. Bollen, K, et al. *Social, Behaviorial, and Economic Sciences Perspectives on Robust and Reliable Science*. National Science Foundation, Arlington, VA, 2015.

9. Begley, CG, et al. Reproducibility in science: improving the standard for basic and preclinical research. *Circulation Research* 2015.

10. Freedman, LP, et al. The economics of reproducibility in preclinical research. *Public Library of Science Biology* 2015.

11. Reichlin, TS, et al. The researcher's view of scientific rigor—survey on the conduct and reporting of *in vivo* research. *Public Library of Science One*. https://doi.org/10.1371.pone.0165999

12. Kilkenny, C, et al. Improving bioscience research reporting: the ARRIVE guidelines for reporting animal research. *Public Library of Science Biology* 2010. https://doi.org/10.1371/journal.pbio.100412

13. Hirsch, C, et al. In vitro research reproducibility: keeping up high standards. *Frontiers in Pharmacology*. https://doi.org/10.3389/fphar.2019.01484

14. Olsen, A, et al. Toward a global and reproducible science for brain imaging in neurotrauma: the ENIGMA adult moderate/severe traumatic brain injury working group. *Brain Imaging and Behavior* 2020. https://doi.org/10.1007/s11682-020-00313-7

15. Poldrack, RA, et al. Scanning the horizon: towards transparent and reproducible neuroimaging research. *Nature Reviews Neuroscience* 2017.

16. Kong, X-Z, Enigma Laterality Working Group, et al. Reproducibility in the absence of selective reporting: an illustration for large-scale brain asymmetry research. *Human Brain Mapping* 2020. https://doi.org/10.1002/hbm.25154

17. Kong, X-Z, et al. Mapping cortical brain asymmetry in 17,141 healthy individuals world-wide via the ENIGMA consortium. *Proceedings of the National Academy of Sciences of the United States of America* 2018.

18. Button, KS, et al. Power failure: why small sample size undermines the reliability of neuroscience. *Nature Reviews Neuroscience* 2013. https://doi.org/10.1038/nrn3475

19. Fanelli, D. "Positive" results increase down the hierarchy of the sciences. *Public Library of Science One*. https://doi.org/10.1371/journal.pone.00168

20. Mobley, A, et al. A survey on data reproducibility in cancer research provides insights into our limited ability to translate findings from the laboratory to the clinic. *Public Library of Science One*. https://doi.org/10.1371/journal.pone.0063221

21. Fanelli, D. Is science really facing a reproducibility crisis, and do we need it to? *Proceedings of the National Academy of Sciences* 2018.

22. Begley, CG, et al. Raise the standards for preclinical research. *Nature* 2012.

23. Prinz, F, et al. Believe it or not: how much can we rely on published data on potential drug targets? *Nature Reviews Drug Discovery* 2011.

24. Errington, TM, et al. An open investigation of the reproducibility of cancer biology research. *eLife* 2014.

25. Baker, M, et al. Reproducibility project yields muddy results. *Nature* 2017.

26. Nosek, B, et al. Making sense of replications. *eLife* 2017. https://doi.org/10.7554/eLife.23383

27. Hardwicke, I, et al. An empirical assessment of transparency and reproducibility-related practices in the social sciences (2014–2017). *Royal Society Open Science* 2020. http://dx.doi.org/10.1098/rsos.190806

28. Camerer, CF, et al. Evaluating the replicability of social science experiments in nature and science between 2010 and 2015. *Nature Human Behavior* 2018.

29. Simmons, JP, et al. False-positive psychology: undisclosed flexibility in data collection and analysis allows presenting anything as significant. *Psychological Science* 2011. https://doi.org/10.1177/09567976|1417632

30. Makel, M, et al. Replications in psychology research: how often do they really occur? *Perspectives on Psychological Science* 2012. https://doi.org/10.1171/1745691612460688

31. Polanin, JR, et al. Transparency and reproducibility of meta-analyses in psychology: a meta-review. *Perspectives on Psychological Science*. https://doi.org/10.1177/1745691620906

32. Open Science Collaboration. "Estimating the reproducibility of psychological science." *Science*. https://doi.org/10.1126/science.aac4716

33. Gilbert, DT, et al. Comment on "Estimating the reproducibility of psychological science." *Science* 2016. https://doi.org/10.1126/science.aad7243

34. Anderson, CJ, et al. Response to comment on "Estimating the reproducibility of psychological science." *Science* 2016;351(6277)1037c,

35. Bressan, P Confounds in "failed" replications. *Frontiers in Psychology* 2019. https://doi.org/10.3389/fpsyg.2019.01884

36. Bohannon, J. Replication effort provokes praise—and "bullying" charges. *Science* 2014.https://doi.org/10.1126/science.344.6186.788

37. Fiske, ST A Call to Change Science's Culture of Shaming. 2016 APS Observer. https://psychologicalscience.org/observer/a-call-to-change-sciences-culture-of-shaming

38. Web of Science, accessed October 10, 2020.

39. Sherry, CE, et al. Assessment of transparent and producibility research practices in the psychiatry literature. *General Psychiatry* 2020. https://doi.org/10.1136/gpsych-2019-100149

40. Tajika, A, et al. Replication and contradiction of highly cited research papers in psychiatry: 10-year follow-up. *British Journal of Psychiatry* 2015. https://doi.org/10.1192/bjp.bp.113.143701

41. Fried, EI, et al. The 341 737 ways of qualifying for the melancholic specifier. *Lancet Psychiatry* 2020.

42. Fried, DI, et al. Depression is not a consistent syndrome: an investigation of unique symptom profiles in the STAR*D study. *Journal of Affective Disorders* 2012.

43. Kochunov, P, et al. Toward high reproducibility and accountable heterogeneity in schizophrenia research. *JAMA Psychiatry* 2019. https://doi.org/10.1001/jamapsychiatry.2019.0208

44. Zachar, P, et al. The aspirations for a paradigm shift in DSM-5: an oral history. *Journal of Nervous and Mental Disease* 2019.

45. Alnæs, D, et al. Brain heterogeneity in schizophrenia and its association with polygenic risk. *JAMA Psychiatry* 2019. https://doi.org/10.1001/jamapsychiatry.2019.0257. Corrected on July 17, 2019.

46. Blackford, JU. Leveraging statistical methods to improve validity and reproducibility of research findings. *JAMA Psychiatry* 2017. https://doi.org/10.1001/jamapsychiatry.2016.3730

47. Acheson, A, et al. Reproducibility of tract-based white matter microstructural measures using the ENIGMA-DTI protocol. *Brain and Behavior* 2017. https://doi.org/10.1002/brb3.615

48. Maïza, O, et al. Reproducibility of fMRI activations during a story listening task in patients with schizophrenia. *Schizophrenia Research* 2011;128(1–3):98–101. https/doi.org/10.1016/j.schres.2011.01.025.

49. Koshiyama, D, et al. Neuroimaging studies with cognitive genetics collaborative research organization aiming to replicate and extend works of ENIGMA. *Human Brain Mapping* 2020. https://doi.org/10.1002/hbm.25040

50. Frégnac, Y. Big data and the industrialization of neuroscience: a safe roadmap for understanding the brain? *Science* 2017;358(6362):470–492.

51. Bell, V. Open science in mental health research. *Lancet Psychiatry* 2017. http://dx.doi.org/10.1006/52215-0366(17)30244-4

52. Fanelli, D. Is science really facing a reproducibility crisis, and do we need to? *Publication of the National Academy of Science* 2018. www.pnas.org/gi/doi/10.1037/pnas.1708272114

# 8

# Distorted Outcomes and Retractions
## *Prevalence and Types*

## Introduction

There is no doubt that the massive increase in the number of journals and articles has made it difficult for clinicians and others involved in the health care system to read and incorporate the results of research into their practices and organizational decisions. The growth of meta-analytic studies from almost zero in the early 1990s to 11,000 in 2017[1] has helped to summarize the results of some 20 million articles available at the start of this century.[2] Unfortunately, meta-analyses have their own deficits,[1] as we explored in Chapter 6. An additional time-saving route for busy clinicians, students, historians, and journalists, involves skipping the body of the text, and focusing on the abstract and conclusions of individual studies. That being the case, it is clear that investigators have an obligation to ensure the accuracy of those sections, but the evidence suggests a number of serious problems, as we shall see. Making matters worse, the evidence also suggests that the number of retractions in the scientific literature is increasing, leaving clinicians, patients, and organizations even more uncertain about the validity of studies, further compromising the risk–benefit ratio and rational prescribing.

## Study outcomes

In 2016, the *Journal of Clinical Epidemiology* published[3] an analysis of 190 Cochrane and non-Cochrane systematic reviews or meta-analyses from the year 2010. The search revealed 2,328 studies in that year alone, but a series of filters left only190. The primary goal of the study: to evaluate the frequency with which the reviews reported the absolute effect size of the benefits and harms, as well as the relative effect size. Reporting of both the absolute and relative effect sizes is recommended by the Preferred Reporting Items for Systematic Reviews and Meta-Analyses (PRISMA).[4] We should stress that the absolute effect size is the more important for clinical decision making, since the relative effect size can result in an inflated estimate of what the treatment can accomplish. The relative effect size can also exaggerate small, between-group differences for uncommon events, and minimize larger differences for common events. The authors noted that absolute measures of interest include the number needed to treat (NNT), the risk difference (RD), and the proportion of harmful or beneficial events in groups. Relative measures include the risk or rate ratio (RR), odds ratio, hazard ratio, and relative risk reduction.

Despite the advantages of citing absolute effect sizes, only 22.5% of reviewed abstracts reported the absolute effects size when addressing benefits.[3] Even fewer, 12.8%, cited the absolute risk for harms. When considering harm overall, 38% reported critically important outcomes of harm in the full text, but, of the 38%, only 63% reported these in the abstract!

Important outcomes of harm were noted in 51% of the texts, while 69% reported them in the abstracts. There were no reporting differences in the Cochrane vs non-Cochrane Reviews. The authors concluded that investigators often did not report the most patient-important outcomes with regard to benefits and harms in their abstracts and summaries, potentially clouding the risk–benefit ratio.

The authors cited several studies that found similar results, including an evaluation[5] of 344 articles on health inequalities published in the top 4 journals in medicine and the top 4 public health journals in 2009. Only 138 of the 344 articles cited numeric data in the abstract, with 9% reporting an absolute measure, 88% a relative measure of effect, and only 2% reporting both. Yet the authors held out hope that matters will improve, given the publication of the PRISMA guidelines in 2013.[4]

Despite such hope, Parsons et al.[6] reported in 2019 that of 1,376 systematic review protocols involving health care interventions, only 38% (524) listed the adverse event outcomes! Of the 524 protocols, 186 were systematic reviews, but 41 were excluded secondary to various problems with access or duplications, leaving 146 systematic reviews for further analysis. Of the 146 systematic reviews, 65% fully reported on adverse events, as required by the protocols. However, 27% partially reported adverse events, or altered the reporting outcomes! Eight percent completely failed to report adverse outcomes, while in 7%, the authors' report of outcomes differed from the protocol. This was done by changing the wording, reporting only grades of severity instead of all adverse outcomes, and failing to designate the event as a primary or secondary outcome.

An earlier paper by Chan et al.,[7] also noted inconsistencies in 122 published outcomes that had been compared with the study protocols in 102 RCTs of health care interventions. (The authors were able to obtain unrestricted access to the trial protocols.) Not surprisingly, studies with statistically significant outcomes were more than twice as likely to fully report on efficacy, and 4.7 times more likely to fully report harms. Overall, 50% of efficacy outcomes and 65% of harms outcomes per trial were incompletely reported. Compared with the protocols, 62% of the published articles had at least one primary outcome that was introduced, omitted, or changed. In other words, the outcomes were changed during analysis of the data, in order to fit the data! This is completely unacceptable, although the authors hedged a bit due to the lack of data on unreported outcomes. Even worse, 86% of survey responders actually denied the existence of unreported outcomes, despite clear evidence, perhaps reflecting concern over the presence of such data.

These results are worrisome at best, and as the authors state, pose a threat to the reliability of the published literature, including meta-analyses.[7, p.2464] Yet a bright spot was found in a 2020 study by Bamat et al.,[8] who found protocol adherence rates of 91.5% in superiority trials and 89.8% of the non-inferiority trials published in three high impact journals.

Another way of altering outcomes involves using surrogate outcomes, rather than well-defined clinically important outcomes. The difference was defined by the Institute of Medicine in 2013,[9] which defined surrogate outcomes as biomarkers intended to substitute for a well-defined and critical clinical endpoint. For example, the investigator can use a decrease in glycosolated haemoglobin levels as surrogates in treatment trials for type II diabetes mellitus, rather than focusing on the more difficult-to-measure outcomes such as vascular complications, poor wound healing, or blindness. This is not to say that glycosolated haemoglobin levels are not important in the management of diabetes mellitus, and indeed can affect the long-term outcomes just mentioned. On the other hand, improvement in surrogate outcomes may not be accompanied by reductions in the overt clinical complications of the disease.[10] Obviously, hard clinical outcomes are vitally important to patients, and are definitive with regard to the course of a disease.[11] In addition, the use of surrogate outcomes has sometimes resulted in treatments ultimately found to be harmful.[12]

Given these concerns, Grey et al.[11] investigated the types of primary outcomes in 416 interventions, as well as sources of sponsorship in 360 RCTs published in 7 major medical journals, and 10 specialty journals in 5 clinical disciplines. (The journals included the *New England Journal of Medicine, Lancet*, and other high-impact journals.) Fifty-six percent of the trials were focused on drugs, 12% on procedures, and 4% on devices, assuring a spectrum of interventions. Despite the concerns over surrogate outcomes, 62% of the primary outcomes were surrogate, with another 50 trials reporting mixed surrogate/hard outcomes, leaving only 24% of trials with a hard, primary outcome. (Hard outcomes included myocardial infarction, stroke, mortality, incident disease, resolution of infections, survival, etc.) Non-industry funding was found in 61% of trials, but the type of journal or source funding were not associated with type of outcome. Note that trials of devices and procedures were infrequently published, despite their place in clinical practice. Clearly, these findings reinforced the concerns raised by Yukdin et al.[10] and Svensson et al.[12]

## Are rates of retractions and research fraud increasing?

In 2012, Fang et al.[13] noted a 10-fold increase in the number of retractions dating from 1975, with most retractions secondary to research misconduct! Another study[14] of articles indexed by PubMed compared the total of indexed articles to the number of retractions during the years 1973–2011. and found nearly a 4-fold increase. Research misconduct had been defined by the United States Office of Science and Technology Policy in 2000 as fabrication, falsification, or plagiarism in reviewing, proposing, reporting, and performing research.[15] Note that the first article retracted for plagiarism had been published in 1979, and the first retraction for duplicate publication appeared in 1990. However, it was not until 2005 that we had the first empirical evidence for the extent of questionable research practices.[16] This came in the form of a confidential survey of 3,600 mid-career scientists who had received their first research grant between 1991 and 2001, and an early-career sample of 4,160 NIH-supported post-doctoral trainees in 2000 or 2001. The response rate varied between 43% and 52%. The survey asked respondents whether they had participated during the previous 3 years in 10 behaviors thought to reflect serious misconduct, including falsification of data, failure to present contradictory data, use of ideas from others without attribution, and unauthorized use of confidential data. Six other behaviors, thought to be less serious, included duplicate publication of data, inappropriate listing of authors, and using inadequate research design.

With regard to the top 10 serious behaviors, 33% of respondents admitted to participating in at least one behavior. Thirty-eight percent of the mid-career scientists acknowledged such behaviors, significantly more than in the early career group. A bright spot: Frequencies of misbehaviors in six of the top 10 categories were under 2%, including falsification and plagiarism. This figure was supported by a systematic review and meta-analysis[17] of 11,647 scientists which found that 2% had committed research fraud in their career. In another survey of 2,212 scientists,[18] the authors cited an incidence rate of 3% per year. Nevertheless, Martinson et al.[16] feared that the data might be under-reported, no doubt secondar to concerns over discovery. (Indeed, as I noted in the introduction to this volume, de Vrieze reported on a study in the Netherlands that 8% of Dutch scientists admitted to research fraud.) Martinson et al.[16] also drew attention to the possibility that simply blaming a few "bad apples" for misconduct actually neglects the role of the research environment in allowing or fostering such behaviors. some of which might stem from perceptions regarding the alleged lack of fairness in grant distributions and resources in general—a topic we shall say more about later.

Although many studies have focused on medical journals, other fields have also been affected. For example, a review[19] of 1582 retracted studies on genetics that had been published from 1970 to 2018, found that 33% had engaged in research misconduct and 24% in duplication of studies, but only 0.8% involved fabrication/falsification and plagiarism, which was more common in non-medical genetic articles. However, medical genetic articles were more likely to be investigated and were retracted sooner. In instances of fabrication/falsification, mean time to retraction was 4.7 years. However, this means that falsified articles were in the literature for almost 5 years! The overall estimated rate of retraction in genetics was estimated at 0.15%, vs estimated retraction rates across fields of 0.02%–0.04.% In a study of retracted surgical papers during 1991–2015, King et al.[20] reviewed 184 articles, primarily from general, cardiac, and orthopedic surgery. Duplication was the most common reason for retraction at 35%, followed by institutional review board violations in 18.5%, falsified data in 14.7%, data errors in 9.8%, and plagiarism in 8.2.% Lower percentages were found for copyright violations, lack of financial disclosures, and consent violations. In an alarming study[21] of data from the Retraction Watch database, the authors noted that the retraction rate of studies involving COVID-19 patients exceeded the basal rate of 4 in 10,000 papers found in earlier research on viral epidemics. The authors also stressed that about 137 articles are appearing daily on the pandemic, raising concerns about the rapid appearance and validity of the results, as I described in the introduction.

## Retractions: Costs and consequences

Beyond the obvious damage to the trust and credibility of science, a practical issue is the cost of retractions. Stern et al.[22] attempted an analysis of the costs by focusing on research sponsored by the National Institutes of Health (NIH), and found that $46.9 million in funds had been expended in the support of 149 studies that were eventually retracted, but this represented only 0.01% of the $451 billion NIH budget between 1992 and 2012. On the other hand, some investigators had not acknowledged their funding sources, so the authors recalculated the costs of 43 articles reporting only NIH funding. This resulted in a cost of $123 million over 20 years, but wait: What if retracted papers comprised only a small sample of papers marked by misconduct? Based on published rates of misconduct, the authors estimated a cost of $12.4 billion, but this was only 1.5% of the NIH research budget, and quite possibly an overestimation. Nevertheless, there are other direct costs, such as the cost of investigations (salaries and legal fees), and indirect costs, including damage to reputations, problems in recruitment, obtaining grants in the future, and decreased productivity. In 35 cases, however, authors of studies cited by the Office of Research Integrity (ORI) actually published more articles yearly *after* the ORI reports.

Another issue: What of the possible harms to patients enrolled in studies that were retracted? In an effort aimed at documenting such risks, Steen[23] examined 788 retracted papers found in the PubMed database covering the years 2000–2010. However, they excluded over 400 basic science studies, case reports, reviews, and those not available on the Web of Knowledge, leaving 180 primary studies. More than 28,000 patients had been enrolled, and 9,189 treated in these primary papers. Retracted papers were cited more than 5,000 times, with 93% of these involving research investigations, in which 400,000 subjects were enrolled, and 70,501 were treated! Worse, 70 studies cited for fraud had treated more patients per study than did papers retracted secondary to errors. While Steen gave us details on several widely cited studies on research harms, he described several limitations to the study, including:

- A lack of information on actual harm, a critical shortcoming;
- All cases of possible harm are not equivalent;
- The number of citations does not necessarily reflect the intellectual/clinical impact of the primary research;
- Obviously, there was no information on harms that came to subjects not enrolled in a study but treated for the same condition, so this vital comparison could not be done;
- The number of retractions is likely an underestimate, due in part to the length of time needed to publish retractions.

As a corollary to this study, we note that there are two types of post-publication citations of retracted papers.[24] These involve citations that articles received *after* retraction, or citations that appeared *prior* to retraction. Are there differences in the rates of the two forms of citations? It appears so. Bar-Ilan and Helevi,[25] in a study of retracted articles that had received more than 10 citations post-publication, found that the great majority were positive, no matter the clear retraction notice by the journal editor, and regardless of the reason for retraction. Obviously, the longer the time to retraction, the greater the odds of it being cited, absent gross fraud. Indeed, during the years 2003–2012, the mean time-to-retraction of 1,595 articles was 33.8 months ($\pm$35.63 SD), significantly longer than the 452 articles published a decade earlier, at 29.60 months ($\pm$28.54 SD).[14]

## Summary[26]

- Retractions have increased over time, but the rate leveled off after 2012.
- The increase appears to be, at least in part, due to the number of journals, editors being more aware of the problem, and adoption of policies aimed at preventing publication of questionable studies. Yet many journals did not report a single retraction after 2003.
- About 500 of 30,000 authors account for about 25% of retractions. One hundred of the 500 each had 13 retractions or more! What is being done to investigate recurrent offenders?
- About half of retractions involve fabrication, falsification, or plagiarism, serious offenses.

Nevertheless, it seems clear that we have more to accomplish, given the long half-life of some retracted papers, the potential harms to patients, and effects on the risk–benefit ratio secondary to erroneous research results. This should be a top priority for institutional review boards, which generally seem to do a good job of protecting harms to potential subjects during the enrollment process, but, so far as I'm aware, do little to investigate the harms from failed or fraudulent studies.

## References

1. deVrieze, J. The metawars. Meta-analyses were supposed to end scientific debates. Often, they only cause more controversy. *Science* 2015.

2. Tajika, A, et al. Replication and contradiction of highly-cited research papers in psychiatry: 10-year follow-up. *British Journal of Psychiatry* 2015.

3. Agarwal, A, et al. Authors seldom report the most patient-important outcomes and absolute effect measures in systematic review abstracts. *Journal of Clinical Epidemiology* 2017. http://dx.doi.org/10.1016/j.clinepi.2016.08.064

4. Beller, EM, et al. PRISMA for abstracts: reporting systematic reviews in journals and conference abstracts. *Public Library of Science Medicine* 2013.

5. King, NB, et al. Use of relative and absolute effect measures in reporting health inequalities: structured review. *British Medical Journal* 2012.

6. Parsons, R, et al. More than one-third of systematic reviews did not fully report the adverse events outcome. *Journal of Clinical Epidemiology* 2019. https://doi.org/10.1016/j.jclinepi.2018.12.007

7. Chan, A-W, et al. Empirical evidence for selective reporting of outcomes in randomized trials. Comparison of protocols to published articles. *JAMA* 2004.

8. Bamat, NA, et al. Protocol adherence rates in superiority and nonferiority randomized clinical trials published in high impact medical journals. *Clinical Trials*. Early access July 2020.

9. Institute of Medicine 2010. Evaluation of biomarkers and surrogate endpoints in chronic disease. http://www.nationalacademies.org/hmd/reports2010/evaluation-of-biomarkers-and-surrogate-endpoints-in-chronic-disease.aspx. Accessed October 17, 2020.

10. Yudkin, JS, et al. The idolatry of the surrogate. *British Medical Journal* 2011.

11. Grey, P, et al. Outcomes, interventions and funding in randomized research published in high-impact journals. *Biomed Central* 2018. https://doi.org/10.1186/s13063-018-2978-8

12. Svensson, S, et al. Surrogate outcomes in clinical trials: a cautionary tale. *JAMA Internal Medicine* 2013.

13. Fang, FC, et al. Misconduct accounts for the majority of retracted scientific publications. *Proceedings of the National Academy of Sciences* 2012.

14. Steen, RG, et al. Why has the number of scientific retractions increased? *Public Library of Science One* 2013. https://doi.org/101371/journal.pone.0068397

15. OSTP Federal Policy on Research Misconduct. http://www.ostp.gov/html/001207.html (2005)

16. Martinson, BC, et al. Scientists behaving badly. *Nature* 2005.

17. Fanelli, D. How many scientists fabricate and falsify research? A systematic review and meta-analysis. *Public Library of Science One* 2009.

18. Titus, SL, et al. Repairing research integrity. *Nature* 2008.

19. Dal-Ré, F, et al. Reasons for and time to retraction of genetics articles published between 1970 and 2018. *Journal of Medical Genetics* 2019. https://doi.org/10.1136/jmedgenet-2019-106137

20. King, EG, et al. Analysis of retracted articles in the surgical literature. *American Journal of Surgery* 2018.

21. Yeo-The, NSL, et al. An alarming retraction rate for scientific publications on coronavirus disease. *Accountability in Research* 2019. https://doi.org/10.1080/08989621.2020.1782203

22. Stern, AM, et al. Research: financial costs and personal consequences of research misconduct resulting in retracted publications. *Elifesciences* 2014. https://doi.org/10.7554/eLife.02956.001

23. Steen, RG. Retractions in the medical literature: how many patients are put at risk by flawed research? *Journal of Medical Ethics* 2011. https://doi.org/10.1136/jme.2011.043133

24. Unger, K, et al. Even retracted papers endure. *Science* 2006.

25. Bar-Ilan, J, et al. Post-retraction citations: a case study. *Scientometrics* 2017;113:547–565. https://doi.org/10.1007/s11192-017-2242-0

26. Brainard, JJ. Rethinking retractions. *Science* 2018;363(6413):390–395.

# 9

# Journalology, Predatory Journals, Peer Review, Pre-Prints, and Guidelines

## Introduction

In previous chapters, we have stressed the adverse effects of money and Big Pharma on medical science, although in some instances the gains have been positive. However, the wealth of Pharma and the remarkable growth of the research establishment have been accompanied by an exponential growth of publications and journals, reaching some 20 million articles and 5,000 journals by the year 2000.[1] This has resulted in a rapid increase in systematic reviews and meta-analytic studies aimed at answering important clinical questions. Yet, as we have seen in Chapter 6, meta-analyses have had their own problems, including bias and inconsistent results. Adding to the problems facing clinicians who wish to prescribe rationally, the literature has become subject to contamination by the development of predatory, for-profit journals that have increased from 59 in 2012[2] to at least 1,350 today.[3] Adding to the mix of information, we now have the Directory of Open Access Journals (DOAJ) that listed 8,250 journals in 2012. Some of these are these are considered credible,[2] but this may not be true in all cases, as shall see in a moment. The proliferation of journals, some without editorial boards or sufficient peer review, has led to the development of multiple guidelines and regulations aimed at rapid publication, but compliance has been an ongoing problem, as we will see shortly.

## Predatory journals

The rise of predatory journals began in 2012, as documented by Jeffrey Beall at the University of Colorado.[3] Beall observed that such journals were defined by undisclosed fees, unprofessional practices, and poor English. Other flaws[4] have included solicitation of papers by websites and emails, many of which promote rapid publication on receipt of a high publication fee. Since the journals have little or no peer review or editorial boards, papers are often guaranteed publication, a tempting pitch indeed, given the pressure to publish and obtain promotions and grants. Adding to the temptation is the possibility of presenting one's work at national or international conferences that do not meet scientific expectations, but are gaining in popularity, and, according to one study,[5] now outnumber official scholarly events.

Alarmed by the growth of predatory journals and publishers, a staff investigator, John Bohannon, a staff writer with the journal *Science*,[2] concocted a deeply flawed scientific paper which he sent to 304 open-access journals, 167 journals listed by the DOAJ, 121 from Beall's list of predatory journals, and to 16 listed by Beall and the DOAJ. The paper had been slightly modified in order to avoid detection by reviewers and labeled as a duplicate submission. Of the 304 open-access journals, 157 accepted it, but only 36 of the 157 acknowledged the scientific

DOI: 10.1201/9781003267218-10

flaws. Remarkably, 45% of the journals listed in the DOAJ accepted it, including several journals published by top-tier companies such as Elsevier, Wolters Kluwer, and Sage. Although they accepted his fake paper, they did take corrective action after Bohannon contacted them following their acceptance. Bohannon also described other problems within the predatory journal world, including falsifying geographical locations, abandoning websites, providing wrong addresses, and demanding that the author pay a publication fee for submission.[2]

Bohannon concluded with the obvious: That many open-access publishers are failing to do adequate peer review, and that journals without quality control standards are destructive to science generally, not to speak of clinicians and patients. Nevertheless, even top-tier journals continue to have problems.[6] For example, Godlee et al.,[7] wrote an article with eight deliberate mistakes and sent it to 200 regular reviewers of the *British Medical Journal*. No reviewer spotted all of the mistakes, and most reported fewer than two.

These concerns are not new, and have prompted multiple efforts to improve matters, as summarized by Couzin-Frankel.[6] In 1989, the first Peer Review Congress met in Chicago, with 300 attendees and 50 abstracts. This was the start of Journalology as a scientific field. In 1996, the Consolidated Standards of Reporting Trials (CONSORT) were published and were periodically updated. By 2018, CONSORT had been endorsed by 585 journals. Despite these corrective efforts, an editorial published in 2020[4] cited studies indicating that 25% of all journals may be predatory, and that this segment of the journal world has been valued at some $10 billion, a figure that almost certainly will grow, given the popularity of predatory journals.[3]

## The impact of predatory journals

While the overall impact remains to be seen, Wilkinson et al.[8] noted the pervasiveness of what they described as academic spam emails sent from predatory journals to career development grant awardees at the NIH. Queries were sent to the awardees in 2016, asking about the frequency of such emails and how they responded to them. Fifty-four percent had received from 1 to 10 spam emails daily, and had spent from 1 to 10 minutes daily evaluating them. Interestingly, time spent in evaluating the emails was correlated with publishing in an open-access format, and the number of articles published in peer-reviewed journals. The awardees acknowledged a sense that they could be missing career opportunities by ignoring the emails. This alarmed the authors, who emphasized the need to address the problem as quickly as possible.

More support for an urgent corrective strategy can be found in a study[9] of applicants for faculty positions at a pharmacology school. The applicants appeared to inflate their collective publication record of 1,020 papers by including 181 papers published in predatory journals. The applicants further claimed that they had served on 141 editorial boards, but 64.5% of the boards were affiliated with publishers of predatory journals. Remarkably, 22% of the applicants had at least half of their articles printed in such journals! We should note too that the allure of predatory journals is not limited to the United States, with India serving as the largest base for open access publishing.[2] Indeed, Bohannon noted[2] that only 15 journals based in India rejected his flawed paper, while 64 accepted it. In South Africa, a decision by the government to award academics a prize of $7,000 for each paper published[10] led to a 140% increase in papers published by predatory journals!

The lure of predatory journals has spread to the COVID-19 era, as documented by Vervoort et al.,[11] who analyzed 833 journals found in Beall's list, and another site, Stop Predatory Journals. Verfoort et al. searched for articles containing the terms corona virus, COVID-19, and SARS-CoV-2 published during the months of January to May 2020. The authors found 125 original articles, 172 reviews, and 70 commentaries published in 114 predatory journals.

Article processing charges were estimated at US$46,057. After excluding a few journals due to uncertainty regarding the charges, the processing charges came to US$33,807 for 350 articles. While Vervoort et al. did not investigate the publication content, they did comment, as have others, on the use of scripted emails to enlist authors, and the presence of publication fees, which averaged some US$98.00, an amount that might disproportionately affect investigators in lower-income countries. Beyond the financial issues, the authors cited other several major concerns from this practice, including the loss of biomedical and epidemiological information, and the spread of misinformation with potentially harmful consequences, as found in articles that touted the efficacy of homeopathy for COVID-19. (Other problems with articles on the pandemic were cited in the Introduction, and more will be describe later in this chapter.)

There is no doubt that predatory journals and conferences have spread across multiple fields and countries, as a visit to the Web of Science[12] on October 26, 2020 confirmed. I queried the site for articles on predatory journals published in the past 5 years, and received 554 hits, citing their presence in radiology, anesthesiology, economics, and other areas. Predatory journals were found in countries ranging from Brazil and Canada to Latin America, Malaysia, Pakistan and South Africa. Whether knowingly or not, hundreds of scientists have served as peer reviewers for predatory journals,[13] while articles published in predatory journals are finding their way into standard databases such as PubMed.[14]

## What constitutes a predatory journal?

Despite these findings, some have noted that there is no formal agreement on how to define a predatory journal, and no set of operationalized criteria[15] useful for a definition. That being the case, the authors first developed a set of questions regarding definitions, educational outreach, policy initiatives, and technological solutions that might aid in stopping submissions. Surveys were then sent to selected experts in the field. After the responses were obtained, a summit conference was held in order to integrate the responses and suggestions. Of the proposed seven markers that might be useful in identifying predatory journals, a consensus was reached on three:

- The use of aggressive/persuasive emails in soliciting articles
- Contact details of the publisher are difficult to verify
- The journals lack a retraction policy

Regarding empirically derived data, consensus was reached on the following:

- The journal home page lacks professionalism
- Affiliations of the editors and editorial board are not verifiable
- The journal is not a member of COPE, nor does it mention a Creative Commons license

Other recommendations included additional funding for study of predatory journals, development of a single checklist useful for identification, and more emphasis on education aimed at informing students and faculty on the risks of publishing in predatory journals. In that regard, a "one-stop shop" should be established that would include a repository of training and educational materials. The need for a single checklist is obvious, sine a systematic review[16] in 2020 found 90 checklists, each with a mean of 11 items. However, only three of the checklists met evidence-based criteria. For the busy clinician or investigator, the current checklists provide little assistance in separating legitimate journals from the predatory group.

Yet for all the concerns over the effects of predatory journals on science and clinical practice, one group[17] claimed that the articles published therein pose little threat to science. They based their conclusion on a study of citation frequency garnered by articles published in predatory journals, where they found an average of 2.6 citations per article. Fifty-six percent of the articles were not cited at all. In marked contrast, a random sample of articles in the SCOPUS Index gathered 18.1 citations per article, while only 9% had no citations. As noted above, others disagreed with the authors' conclusion, but at least these findings provide some hope that investigators are being discrete in their choice of journals. Given the ongoing debate, it is interesting that the Federal Trade Commission has joined the fray, filing a lawsuit against OMICS, a company that publishes hundreds of open access journals, after receiving multiple complaints from investigators regarding the lack of peer review and other promised services. In early 2009, a U.S. District Court judge ordered OMICS to pay $50 million in damages.[18]

## Peer review and publications: Problems and solutions

On October 4, 2013, the journal Science published a special section on problems with scientific publishing, noting that in the middle of the 20th century, we had experienced a "key innovation," in science, the anonymous referee.[19] However, the sense of trust that fostered this development has been badly eroded by changes in publication practices, a number of which we have reviewed. It now appears that the aforementioned "key innovation," the anonymous referee, has come under attack. Indeed, one prominent critic, Vitek Tracz, has insisted that the peer-reviewed print journal will cease to exist by 2023.[20] To that end, he founded BioMed Central (BMC) in 2000, an open-access enterprise that in 2013 had some 250 journals in its catalogue. Authors are charged a $500 publishing fee. He then took on anonymous peer review, a process that contains an inherent conflict of interest, since reviewers are often in competition with the studies that they review, a problem that may not only delay publication,[20] but result in the theft of intellectual property. His answer: The introduction in 2013 of F1000Research, an organization that publishes almost immediately after receipt and a short quality check. This seems a daunting process, since authors must include the entire data set. Only then does peer review occur. The reviewers must post their names and affiliations with their critiques, and, in marked contrast to the standard peer-review format, the process does not stop with acceptance by the journal, but results in an ongoing dialogue between authors and reviewers.

Does this appeal to authors, many of whom are already dealing with significant demands on their time? While the F1000Research approach is an intriguing development, one notes a counter-argument by Harley[21] in the same issue of Science. Harley cites empirical research indicating that scholars are not enthusiastic about the promise of a revolution in publication practices based on big data, informatics, and algorithms. Instead, authors are choosing journals based on advancing their career self-interests, especially when seeking promotion and tenure. This means relying on peer-reviewed publications in highly regarded journals with high visibility. Nevertheless, the shift to open access continues, with the Howard Hughes Medical Institute[22] requiring in 2020 that its staff scientists immediately make their papers free to read by publishing in open-access journals, or by putting papers in a near-final, peer-reviewed form in a freely accessible archive. The Nature group of journals in 2021 will require[23] that scientists in German research institutes be free to publish an unlimited number of articles in no-fee journals that are open to all readers. Funding will be provided by institutional payments to the journals, at an estimated cost of $11,200 per article.

What else can be done to improve peer-review, publication practices, and the validity of the literature? The *British Medical Journal* (*BMJ*)[24] has called for more research and better funding of studies on peer review and the publication process, areas in which the *BMJ* has been quite active, having published a number of such studies. The *BMJ* also sponsors the Peer Review Congress, along with *JAMA*, the *JAMA* Network, and the Meta-Research Innovation Network.[24] The ninth meeting of the Peer Review Congress is scheduled for 2022, with calls for papers on bias, peer-review, decision-making, research and publication ethics, quality, models for peer review, and better dissemination of information.[25] Other relevant governmental organizations[26] in the United States include the Office of Scientific Integrity (OSI), established within the NIH in 1989 with the goal of investigating scientific fraud. In 1992, the OSI moved to the Public Health service, and was renamed the Office of Research Integrity (ORI), while the National Science Foundation developed an Office of the Inspector General.

## Sharing and dissemination of information

In 2018, The International Committee of Medical Journal Editors (ICMJE) strongly recommended that ICMJE journals, and their affiliated journals, commit to a data-sharing policy in order to improve research, development, and the integrity of science. Yet a study[27] of 100 RCTs from each set of journals revealed that only 35% of member journals and 30% of affiliated journals had an explicit data-sharing policy on their websites. Nevertheless, 77% of RCTs in the member journals explicitly noted that data sharing was an objective, as opposed to 25% of the affiliated journals. The authors suggested that ongoing audits could enhance compliance. Similar results were found in a study[28] of the Consolidated Standards of Reporting Trials (CONSORT),[29] which had recommended in 1996 that the results of RCTs be accompanied by a discussion of *all* available evidence, including systematic reviews, in an effort to improve the clarity and completeness of RCTs. Yet when Clarke and Chalmers[28] examined the discussion sections of 26 RCTs published in 5 general medical journals, only 2 articles included a systematic review of previous evidence. In another four articles, references cited relevant systematic reviews, but there was no attempt to integrate the findings.

In the meantime, a number of investigators have attempted to develop strategies aimed at improving peer review, but the results have not been impressive. For example, Godlee et al.,[7] sent a paper accepted for publication to 420 reviewers, but with modifications that introduced 8 areas of weakness.

The reviewers were randomly allocated into five groups:

*Groups 1 and 2*: Were sent manuscripts in which the authors' names and affiliations were removed.

*Groups 3 and 4*: These reviewers were aware of the authors' identities.

*Groups 1 and 3*: Reviewers were asked to sign their reviews, while groups 3 and 4 returned their reviews unsigned.

*Group 5*: The standard peer-review process was in place, with the authors' identities revealed. The peer review was anonymously.

After all of this work, the groups did not differ in the number of weaknesses detected. However, reviewers who were blinded to the authors' identities were less likely to recommend rejection.

A similar controlled study by van Rooyen et al.,[30] found that blinding and unmasking of reviewers made no difference in the quality of the reviews, recommendations, or the time taken for the review. Yet another controlled trial[31] found no effects of training on the quality of reviews! In an anonymous essay from the *Economist* in 2013,[32] the author cited another study in which 1,500 reviewers were rated by editors of leading journals over a 14-year period, and found that the quality of reviews declined with experience. However, I wonder if technological advances had left some reviewers unprepared. In that case, the journal staff had failed to do its homework.

On the bright side, Chauvin et al.[33] set up a comparative study of reporting accuracy of two groups of reviewers who assessed the reporting accuracy of 119 two-arm, parallel group RCTs. One group of early-career researchers had no prior experience in peer review, but underwent a training period using a CONSORT-based peer-review tool (COBPeer). They then used COBPeer to analyze the extent to which manuscripts included the eight important CONSORT domains, and whether the primary outcome had been switched. In contrast, the second group of reviewers used the standard peer-review process. Those using the COBPeer found a significantly greater number of domains that were accurately classified. A similar study, using a short version of the CONSORT checklist for peer reviewers is now underway, with publication of the protocol in the British Medical Journal Open in 2020.[34] This study will compare the findings of an intervention aimed at a group of peer reviewers who will receive a reminder and explanation about the 10 most important CONSORT domains. The comparison group will be reviewers with no training in the CONSORT domains.

A visit to the Web of Science database on November 4, 2020[35] confirms the importance of the CONSORT Standards, with a list of 444 citations published in the past 5 years. The articles using or mentioning the CONSORT Standards ranged over a substantial area of biomedicine, including rehabilitation medicine, psychiatry, rheumatology, thromboembolic disease, pediatric dentistry, and others. Indeed, a 2020 study[36] of 533 RCTs in dentistry found that endorsement of the CONSORT Standards was linked to improvement in the quality of the RCTs. Nevertheless, deficiencies in reporting of RCTs have persisted, with a study[37] of 1122 RCTS found in PubMed in 2012 noting that 31% did not define the primary outcome, while 45% did not describe the sample size calculation, and 50% did not discuss how concealment was accomplished. This is not acceptable.

## The growth of guidelines for controlled clinical trials

Given the continuing concerns over the quality of RCTs, publication practices, and their effects on clinical recommendations, it is not surprising that guidelines are proliferating. In addition to the CONSORT Standards, we have the following:

- EQUATOR (Enhancing the Quality and Transparency of Research) Network, launched in 2008[38]
- SPIRIT (Standard Protocol Items: Recommendations for Interventional Trials) in 2013[39]
- PRO (Patient Reporting Outcomes)[40]
- SPIRIT-PRO Extension,[41] aimed at improving patient-reporting outcomes by refining the checklists and gathering consensus on the objectives. This study was based on the EQUATOR Network's methodological framework[38]
- PRISMA (Preferred reporting items for systematic reviews and meta-analyses), reported in 2009[42]
- PRISMA-DTA Statement for systematic reviews and meta-analyses of studies on diagnostic test accuracy, in 2018[43]
- Extension of the CONSORT 2010 Statement on the reporting of multi-arm, parallel-group randomized trials, 2019.[44] The earlier guidelines had focused on sequential two-arm trials, but 79% of the trials indexed in PubMed were parallel group trials, with 14% of these involving three groups, and 7% involving four or more groups[44]
- Guidelines International Network in 2012,[45] aimed at developing international standards for clinical practice guidelines

- A checklist for modifying the definition of diseases,[46] in 2017. The authors noted that the definitions of diseases are becoming more inclusive across all medical disciplines, despite the lack of acceptable criteria for determining when or how to widen the boundaries of a specific illness. The authors have proposed an 8-item checklist aimed at bringing some structure into this process
- Although not a guideline, another interesting contribution is the Contributor Roles Taxonomy (Credit),[47] that seek to establish standards for authors listed as contributors

As one can see from the citation list, six of the nine guidelines were published in 2017 or later, so their impact is not clear. This is particularly true with regard to their effects on clinical practice and decision-making by prescribers, as compared with the effects on journals themselves. We have one before-and-after evaluation[48] of the CONSORT STATEMENT on the quality of reporting of RCTs in four high-impact journals. After implementation of CONSORT Standards, there was a clear improvement in the quality score of RCTs, as well as a significant decrease in reports of vague or incomplete reports of allocation concealment.

This is welcome news, but the authors provided no information on the clinical impact, other than to trust that such efforts will minimize bias and facilitate decision-making. Another problem is the growing number of recommendations for clinical trial protocols, but defects in reporting have been common, with a summary in 2020[49] indicating that up to 60% of trials omit, change, or introduce a new primary outcome compared with the outcome in the study protocol. Given that problem, it should not surprise anyone that during the past decade, 1758 recommendations aimed at reporting of trial outcomes were found in 244 eligible documents.[49] This data was compared with 72 candidate items that had been previously developed, leading to the addition of another 62 items for a total of 132 items. However, 40% were not supported by empirical evidence! Remarkably, none of the documents provided any explicit recommendations against the use of any of the 132 items. The lack of substantial evidence is concerning, and leaves trialists with no clear mandate. In addition, it's difficult to imagine how many investigators and clinicians would read or follow 132 recommendations.

## Trial registration

When compared with the sets of complex guidelines noted above, it would seem that registering clinical trials in advance would be a relatively simple step to improving trial outcomes. The move to trial registration approach began in 2004, with a statement from the International Committee of Medical Journal Editors urging registration of all clinical trials.[50] Three years later, Section 801 of the FDA Amendments Act[51] mandated that clinical trials must be registered in ClinicalTrials.gov, and must be accompanied by information on trial methodology. Investigators were also directed to post data on the primary outcome measure within 1 year at the end of data collection, or within 1 year of early termination. Unfortunately, the results were not impressive. A study in 2015[52] found that only 13% of 13,327 trials had posted summary results within 1 year of completion, while only 38% had entered results at any time up to 2013.

However, some felt that ambiguities in the reporting process might be hindering compliance. This resulted in publication of the Final Rule in 2016,[53] a rule that expanded the definition of adverse events, and mandated publication within 30 days of all submitted information. According to the authors, this ended the days of deciding whether or not summary results are worth reporting ... the time to decide whether a trial is worth doing is before the trial is started, not after participants have been put at risk. Yet ClinicalTrials.gov, launched in 2008,[54] did not address the issue of risk to subjects in trials that have gone awry. Indeed, an investigation by Science in 2020[55] found that investigators and the FDA are not required to warn trial participants of possible harms, even if the FDA had determined that a trial was excessively risky or fraudulent. As a long-time member of an institutional review board, I can attest to the fact that subjects are always warned of possible harms and risks prior to signing an informed consent, but the consent document says nothing about a duty to warn if the trial is later found to be deficient, excessively risky, or fraudulent. This omission must be corrected.

In 2017, Zarin et al.[56] summarized the evidence on trial registration and its effects on clinical research as of 2016 by analyzing data from ClinicalTrials.gov, which at that point contained more than 227,000 records. With regard to clinical trials registered between 2012 and 2014, an analysis of 49,751 trials revealed that almost 33% were not registered on time, although the rates varied depending on funding sources. Of the late registrations, a large proportion were registered more than 12 months after the start date! In addition, many entries were incomplete, out of date, or not updated recently. On the other hand, there were only two instances where there were inconsistencies in the published primary outcome measures in the 83 trials with 101 registered primary outcomes.

While ClinicalTrials.gov has about two-thirds of global trial registrations, the authors provided a table of 16 internationally based trial registrations,[56] echoing the growth of guidelines described earlier. Indeed, Europe maintains an EU Clinical Trials Register and an EU Trials Tracker that was set up in 2018.[57] The data is similar, in that only 28% of over 13,000 completed trials had posted their results, violating the rule that requires posting of results within 1 year of trial completion. However, after the development of the Tracker system, compliance improved significantly, but the European Medicines Agency has pushed a new trial registry, the Clinical Trials Information System, which will come online in 2022, and impose new and stricter regulations, which may include legal action for noncompliance. Interestingly, Denmark already has a law that permits fines or imprisonment of offenders, although it has not been invoked!

Another facet of the trial registration picture has to do with the inclusion of registration numbers in abstracts, as recommended by the CONSORT Group.[58] This is sometimes overlooked, but remains important due to the reporting of trials in conference abstracts. In a review of 8 major conferences held in 2017, Wright et al.[59] identified 1546 abstracts that were associated with the term random or randomized, with 1124 reporting results of RCTs. Of these, 64% reported primary results, but only 13% included a trial registration number. Overall, only 34% of the abstracts included at least three of the important CONSORT reporting items.

## What have we learned?

In summary, there is no doubt that serious and repeated attempts have been made in recent years to describe the types and extent of the problems perpetuated and encountered by those doing clinical trials. There is wide agreement that randomized, controlled trials are integral to the foundation from which prescribers gather information useful in balancing the risk–benefit ratios of their treatment recommendations. Yet, as we have seen, serious problems remain with regard to bias, conflicts of interest, peer review, the lure of predatory journals, and a barrage of guidelines, many of which lack solid empirical support. Nevertheless, we must acknowledge the extensive efforts by multiple organizations and investigators to improve matters, including a November 2020 rule[60] by the NIH that requires NIH-funded research projects to share data or explain why not. The data-sharing plan must be present in the publication, or when the grant ends. This is a significant change from a 2003 requirement required data-sharing only in projects that received more than $500,000 yearly in funding.

Adding to the problems in publishing has been the advent of the COVID-19 pandemic, with more than 530,000 relevant papers released by journals or as pre-prints.[61] As we noted in the introduction, the fast-growing mortality rate in the pandemic led to a new urgency with regard to rapid publication of papers on treatment, several of which had to be withdrawn. Nevertheless, the call went out to make more use of pre-prints such as medRxiv, server that made a debut in 2019. Pre-prints offer rapid publication, but with little or no peer review, although steps were taken to develop a rapid form of peer review, but this has not succeeded on a wide scale.[61] However, the number of pre-prints posted by medRxiv increased from 200 on all topics in early 2020 to 2,000 by May of that year, with about 75% focused on COVID-19. A relevant question: How many of the pre-print articles wind up in peer-reviewed journals? Only 5%, as of May 2021, but note that only 0.03% of COVID-19 journal articles have been retracted. In addition, some 77% of these articles have been free to read, considerably higher than the 50% of newly published articles prior to the pandemic, more good news.

## More on open access

A lengthy discussion on the perils and benefits of open access published in 2021 in *Science*[62] provides an overview of these issues. The author notes that 2017 was notable in that articles published in open access exceeded 50% for the first time. On the other hand, Plan S, developed by an international coalition of funders, including the Howard Hughes Medical Institute and the Wellcome Trust, has mandated that its recipients make their articles free to read immediately on publication, effective in January 2021. Yet Plan S has fallen short of expectations, in that it will would apply to only 6% of the papers published across the world in 2017.[62]

In addition, whether open access benefits authors is questionable, since studies have shown that the benefits of increased citations may apply to only 8% of papers, usually so-called "superstar" studies.[62] At the same time, other findings indicate that open access papers may reach a broader audience. Yet the fees charged by open access journals are often quite high. For example, the Nature Research journals charge $11,000 at its top end, and Cell Press, $9,900 for publication in Cell,[62] thus favoring investigators at wealthier and more prominent universities and institutions. Finally, a complete shift to open access might prompt publishers to further increase fees secondary to a decline in subscriptions.

As we have seen in the introduction, and in the next and last chapter, the push for more integrity in science, as exemplified by the CONSORT STANDARDS, the EQUATOR NETWORK, and ClinicalTrials.gov, can be undermined by outright fraud.

# References

1. Takija, A, Ogawa, Y, Takeshima, N, et al. Replication and contradiction of highly-cited research papers in psychiatry: 10-year follow-up. *British Journal of Psychiatry* 2015.
2. Bohannon, J. Who's afraid of peer review? *Science* 2013.
3. Beall, J. Beall's list of potential predatory journals and publishers. Available at: https://beallslist.net/standardalone-journals/. Accessed October 25, 2020.
4. Darbyshire, P, et al. Editorial. Hitting rock bottom: the descent from predatory journals to the predatory PhD. *Journal of Clinical Nursing.* https://doi.org/10.1011/jcn.15516

5. Grove, J. Predatory conferences now outnumber official scholarly events. 2017. https://www.timeshighereducation.com/news/predatory-conferences-now-outnumber-offical-scholarly-events

6. Couzin-Frankel, J. Journals under the microscope. "Journalologists" use scientific methods to study publishing. Is their work improving science? *Science* 2018.

7. Godlee, F, Gale, CR, Martyn, CN. Effect on the quality of peer review of blinding reviewers and asking them to sign their reports: a randomized controlled trial. *JAMA* 1998.

8. Wilkinson, TA, Russell, CJ, Bennett, WE, et al. A cross-sectional survey of predatory publishing emails received by career development grant awardees. *British Medical Journal Open*. 9(5): e027928, 2019.

9. Pond, BB, et al. Faculty applicant's attempts to inflate CVs using predatory journals. *American Journal of Pharmaceutical Education* 2017. https://doi.org/10.3188/jsp.48.3.137

10. Hedding, DW. Payouts push professors toward predatory journals. *Nature* 2019.

11. Vervoort, D, Ma, X, Shrime, MG. Money down the drain: predatory publishing in the COVID-19 era. *Canadian Journal of Public Health* 2020.

12. Web of Science database, accessed October 26, 2020.

13. Van Noorden, R. Hundreds of scientists have peer-reviewed for predatory journals. *Nature* 2020. https://doi.org/10.1038/d41586-202-00709-x

14. Manca, A, et al. How predatory journals leak into PubMed. *Canadian Medical Association Journal* 2018.

15. Cukier, S, et al. Defining predatory journals and the threat they pose: a modified Delphi consensus process. *British Medical Journal Open* 2020. https://doi.org/10.1136/bmjopen-2019-035561

16. Cukier, S, et al. Checklists to detect potential predatory biomedical journals: a systematic review. *BMC Medicine* 2020. https://doi.org.10.1186/s12916-020-01566-1

17. Bjork, B-C, et al. How frequently are articles in predatory open-access journals cited. *Publications* 2020.

18. Publisher must pay damages. *Science* 2019.

19. Stone, R, et al. Scientific discourse: buckling at the seams. *Science* 2013.

20. Rabesandratana, T. The seer of scientific publishing. *Science* 2013.

21. Harley, D. Scholarly communication: cultural contexts, evolving models. *Science* 2013.

22. HHMI mandates open access. *Science* 2020.

23. Brainard, J. Nature journals ink open-access deal. *Science* 2020.

24. Schroter, S, et al. Research in peer review and biomedical publication. *British Medical Journal* 2020. https://doi.org/10.1136/bmj.m661

25. Ioannidis, JPA, et al. The Ninth International Congress on Peer Review and Scientific Publication. *JAMA* 2019.

26. Gross, C. Scientific misconduct. *Annual Review of Psychology* 2015. https://doi.org/10.1146/annurev-psych-122414-033437

27. Siebert, M, et al. Data-sharing recommendations in biomedical journals and randomized controlled trials: an audit of journals following the ICMJE recommendations. *British Medical Journal Open* 2020.

28. Clarke, M, et al. Discussion sections in reports of controlled trials published in general medical journals. *JAMA* 1998.

29. Begg, C, Cho, M, Eastwood, S, et al. Improving the reporting of randomized controlled trials. The CONSORT statement. *JAMA* 1996.

30. Van Rooyen, S, et al. Effect of open peer review on quality of review and on reviewers' recommendations: a randomized trial. *British Medical Journal* 1999. https://doi.org/11.1136/bmj.318.7125.23987828

31. Schroter, S, et al. Effects of training on quality of peer review: randomized controlled trial. *British Medical Journal* 2004.

32. Trouble at the lab. *Economist* 2013, October 19.

33. Chauvin, A, et al. Accuracy in detecting inadequate research reporting by early career peer reviewers using an online CONSORT-base peer-review tool (COBPeer) versus the usual peer review process: a cross-sectional diagnostic study. *BiomedCentral Medicine* 2019. https://doi.org/10.1186/s12916-019-1436-0

34. Speich, B, et al. Impact of the short version of the CONSORT checklist for peer reviewers to improve the reporting of randomized controlled trials published in biomedical journals: a study protocol of a randomized controlled trial. *British Medical Journal Open* 2020. https://doi.org/10.1136/bmjopen-2019-035114

35. Web of Science database, accessed November 4, 2020.

36. Sarkis-Onofre, R, et al. CONSORT endorsement improves the quality of reports of randomized clinical trials in dentistry. *Journal of Clinical Epidemiology* 2020.

37. Odutayo, A, et al. Association between trial registration and positive study findings: cross-sectional study (epidemiological study of randomized trials—ESCORT). *British Medical Journal* 2017.

38. Altman, DG, et al. EQUATOR: reporting guidelines for health research. *Lancet* 2008.

39. Chan, A-W, et al. SPIRIT 2013 statement: defining clinical protocol items for clinical trials. *Annals of Internal Medicine* 2013.

40. Doward, LC, et al. Patient reported outcomes: looking beyond the label claim. *Health and Quality of Life Outcomes* 2000.

41. Calvert, M, et al. Guidelines for inclusion of patient-reported outcomes in clinical trial protocols. The SPIRIT-PRO extension. *JAMA* 2018. https://doi.org/10.1001/jama.2017.21903

42. Moher, D, et al. PRISMA group. Preferred reporting items for systematic reviews and meta-analyses: the PRISMA statement. *Journal of Clinical Epidemiology* 2009.

43. McInnes, MDF, et al. Preferred reporting items for a systematic review and meta-analysis studies on the accuracy of diagnostic test accuracy studies. The PRISMA-DTA statement. *JAMA* 2018. https://doi.org/10.1001/jama.2017.19163

44. Juszcak, E, et al. Reporting of multi-arm parallel-group randomized trials. Extension of the CONSORT 2010 statement. *JAMA* 2019. https://doi.org/10.1001/jama.2019.3087

45. Qaseem, A, et al. Guidelines international network: toward international standards for clinical practice guidelines. *Annals Internal Medicine* 2012.

46. Doust, J, et al. Guidance for modifying the definitions of diseases. A checklist. *JAMA Internal Medicine* 2017. https://doi.org/10.1001/jamainternmed.2017.1302.

47. Brand, A, et al. Beyond authorship: attribution, contribution, collaboration, and credit. *Learn Publications* 2015.

48. Moher, D, et al. For the CONSORT Group. Use of the CONSORT statement and quality of reports of randomized trials. A comparative before-and-after evaluation. *JAMA* 2001.

49. Butcher, NJ, et al. Outcome reporting recommendations for clinical trial protocols and reports: a scoping review. *Trials* 2020. https://doi.10.1186/s13063-020-04440-w

50. De Angelis, C, et al. Clinical trial registration: a statement from the International Committee of Medical Journal Editors. *New England Journal of Medicine* 2004.

51. *Food and Drug Administration Amendments Act of 2007.* Public Law No. 110-85§ 801-007.

52. Anderson, J, et al. Compliance with results reporting at ClinicalTrials.Gov. *New England Journal of Medicine* 2015.

53. Zarin, DA, et al. Trial reporting in ClinicalTrials.Gov—the final rule. *New England Journal of Medicine* 2016.

54. Zarin, DA, et al. The clinical.gov results database—update and key issues. *New England Journal of Medicine* 2011.

55. Piller, C. Official inaction. A science investigation shows that FDA oversight of clinical trials is lax, slow-moving, and secretive and that enforcement is declining. *Science* 2020.

56. Zarin, DA, et al. Update on trial registration 11 years after the ICMJE policy was established. *New England Journal of Medicine* 2017.

57. Casassus, B. European law could boost clinical trials reporting. *Science* 2021.

58. Hopewell, S, et al. CONSORT GROUP. CONSORT for reporting randomized controlled trials in journal and conference abstracts: explanation and elaboration. *Public Library of Science Medicine* 2008. https://doi.org/10.1371/journal.pmed.0050020

59. Wright, EC, et al. Inclusion of clinical trial registration numbers in conference abstracts and conformance of abstracts to CONSORT guidelines. *JAMA Internal Medicine* 2019.

60. Brainard, J. NIH finalizes data-sharing rule. *Science* 2020.

61. Brainerd, J. A COVID-19 publishing revolution? Not yet. *Science* 2021.

62. Brainerd, J. Open access takes flight. *Science* 2021.

# 10

# Can Misconduct and Fraud Be Fixed?

## Introduction

There is no doubt that various forms of scientific misconduct and fraud have long been with us, as described by Broad and Wade in 1982,[1] Goodstein in 1991,[2] and Judson in 2004.[3] These authors and others[4] alleged misconduct by Ptolemy of Alexandria, Isaac Newton, Gregor Mendel, Robert Millikan, and William Summerlin, to name a few. Charles Gross, in his long review of scientific misconduct,[4] writes that the first formal discussion of the problem occurred in 1830, when Charles Babbage cited hoaxing, forging, trimming, and data cooking as prime examples of scientific misconduct. Forgery continued to be a subject of intense concern as the years passed, as was cooking and trimming the data to achieve a desired outcome. In 1996, the National Science Foundation[5] defined misconduct as involving fabrication, falsification, and plagiarism. However, other, more subtle instances of behaviors inimical to the integrity of science have received attention in recent years, including publication bias, lack of reproducibility and replication, misattribution of authorship, lack of transparency, and inadequate or absent peer review, all of which we have examined in previous chapters.

## The Early 1980s: How Did Science Respond?

In his essay on scientific misconduct, Gross[4] gave us a summary of a congressional hearing on fraud in biomedical research that was held in the spring of 1981 by the Investigations and Oversight Subcommittee of the House Science and Technology Committee. The chair noted at the outset that a crucial question centered on whether the reported cases were passing episodes, or whether the culture was creating incentives that were making these cases the tip of an iceberg—a question applicable to the present. In their testimony, the director of the NIH and the president of the National Academy of Sciences clearly opted f aor the first explanation, insisting that the problem of fraud had been grossly exaggerated, and insisted that it occurred very rarely. In addition, they claimed that such behavior was an internal matter that should be handled by the scientific community—although science had no formal procedures for dealing with misconduct. In addition, some on the committee to expressed surprise that the witnesses did not accept the proposition that ethical problems in science might be a legitimate subject for congressional oversight.

As Gross notes,[4] Congress proceeded to pass legislation that required the Secretary of Health and Human Services to develop regulations that would require awardee institutions to develop an administrative process aimed at reviewing cases of scientific fraud, and report them to the Secretary if they were considered substantial. We had cited earlier in this volume the next step, which was the establishment of the Office of Scientific Integrity (OSI) within

DOI: 10.1201/9781003267218-11

the NIH in 1989. In 1992, the OSI became the Office of Research Integrity (ORI) in the Public Health Service.

Although the witnesses in the congressional hearings asserted that that misconduct and fraud were rare, was this correct? Some 10 years later, a survey[6] of 99 universities found that almost half of the faculty and students reported knowledge of several types of misconduct, while 10% claimed that they had personal knowledge of data fabrication. Similarly, in 1992, a survey[7] of research students at a major university found that 11% claimed to have first-hand knowledge of scientists falsifying or fabricating data. Other surveys reviewed by Gross[4] reported even higher rates of misconduct or outright fraud. For example, in a survey[8] of members of the American Association for the Advancement of Science, 27% said they had witnessed fabricated, falsified, or plagiarized data over a decade. On the other hand, in a systematic review and meta-analysis of 21 surveys by Fanelli et al.,[9] only 2% of scientists reported that they had falsified or fabricated data, while 14.2% reported that other scientists had indulged in similar misconduct. In addition, up to 33.7% admitted to a number of other questionable research practices, including bias, carelessness, and data cooking, but up to 72% said they were aware of such questionable behaviors by others! Fanelli[9] concluded that these data most likely underestimated the extent of misconduct.

Here are several more examples. A survey,[10] done in 2000, found that almost 6% of respondents admitted to some form of misconduct, with 4% stating they would cook the data if it would aid in obtaining a grant. Rahman and Ankier, in an essay published in 2020,[11] cited this survey[10] as the only investigation into misconduct in the United Kingdom, in contrast to the United States. For example, Rahman and Ankier[11] summarized three studies (published from 2016 to 2018) examining the publication records of applicants for neurosurgery, ophthalmology, and urology residency programs in the United States, and found that rates of misrepresentation or fabrication of articles ranged from 5% to 45%. In 2019, over 90% of health care education investigators, responding to an international survey,[12] admitted to participating in some form of misconduct, quite the contrast to the optimism generated by the congressional witnesses in 1981. Another survey,[13] of 2,000 scientists in the United States funded by the NIH found a wide range of practices that might affect research integrity. These included:

- Failure to discuss contradictory findings: 5–6%
- Publishing redundant articles: 3–6%
- Inaccurate record keeping: 27%
- Circumventing recruitment practices: 6–9%
- Cooking the data: <1%, a bright spot

Although we discussed retractions earlier, it is worth mentioning that Resnik and Dinse[14] noted that 73% of retractions were related to error, but almost 27% were secondary to fabrication, falsification, or plagiarism, echoing Babbage. Despite the many attempts at cleaning up the literature, these rates increased over time. Indeed, in 2017, Miriam Schuchman published an essay[15] in the Canadian Medical Association Journal stressing that it was time to stop the slide to research fraud, citing the work by Fanelli that we discussed earlier, while adding several other examples of investigators excluding data that had failed to support the desired result.

## Training and Oversight: Helpful?

In Chapter 9, we reviewed the many efforts at improving the integrity of journals and RCTS, including the CONSORT Standards, the Peer Review Congress, the COBPeer tool, EQUATOR, SPIRIT, PRISMA and their extensions, Guidelines International Network,

ClinicalTrials.gov, and a number of trial registries. But these efforts usually involve experienced investigators who are publishing the results of their work. Had they been trained in the research ethics early on? As Shuchman[15] and others[16] have noted, education *prior* to entering the lab has often been seen as a key to preventing misconduct, but have these efforts worked? The evidence so far is not reassuring. For example, the Cochrane Collaboration reviewed[17] 33 articles published in 2001–2009 that measured the effects of interventions thought to have an impact on research integrity and responsible conduct. We should first note that the participants (9,571) came from the ranks of academic faculty, undergraduates, and postgraduates across disciplines and countries. Fifteen of the studies were RCTs, and nine were before-and-after studies. What were the results?

The interventions varied widely, with face-to-face lectures, online lectures, discussion groups, and other activities, but most studies did not use any standardized or validated outcome measures, such that it was impossible to synthesize the findings or do a meta-analysis. Several studies had found positive effects on attitudes regarding plagiarism, but no studies focused on fabrication or falsification. There was a high risk of bias, even in the RCTs, and the overall quality of studies was very low. The magnitude of the interventions was generally small, and positive effects were short-lived. The conclusion: The evidence is uncertain with regard to the effects of training. This is consistent with other studies by Kornfield[18] and Phillips et al.[19]

In another effort to clarify the roots of misconduct, Satalkar and Shaw[20] noted studies indicating that individuals develop their own views on honesty, fairness, and integrity prior to becoming a scientist—a truism to be certain, and one which is self-evident. However, these early experiences may vary considerably, as is obvious when one considers the behavior of psychopaths and narcissists. (I have seen no studies addressing the prevalence of these disorders in scientists.) That being the case, the authors developed a qualitative study of 33 investigators in life sciences and medicine in Switzerland, with the goal of understanding their experiences with regard to research integrity.[20] This was first study to do so. The seniority level among the researchers ranged from junior to mid-level to full professors. Eight worked exclusively in lab settings; eleven were women. All participants signed informed consent. Ten were interviewed in person; the rest by phone or skype. Steps were taken to insure anonymity. Results?

- Two-thirds had not had any formal training, and most had limited awareness of such opportunities. (Formal training is not required in Switzerland.)
- Almost half viewed their early education and upbringing as critical to their sense of integrity.
- Eleven noted that their innate personality traits/character influenced their ideas about research integrity.
- However, the research environment can push the investigator down different paths.
- Thirteen agreed that research integrity should be taught, starting with undergraduate courses, but, in any case, investigators must have some degree of innate honesty.
- Five believed that investigators either have integrity or not, regardless of training.

I might add that given the present sociopolitical climate in the United States, the integrity of our research efforts may well be at additional risk. But the problems are not limited to the United States. For example, a report[21] from the United Kingdom noted that 25% of universities had failed to comply with research integrity guidelines issued in 2012. This report also cited a BBC investigation that found some 300 allegations of research misconduct in 23 of 24 Russell Group Universities in the UK between 2011 and 2016.

With regard to the failure of universities in the UK, we should note that the Cochrane Review[17] found *no interventions aimed at the organizational level* (italics mine). Yet as

**85**

recently as 2019, a report[22] in *Nature* noted an "epic case of research fraud" perpetrated by a now-deceased investigator who had carried out his work at four universities in the United States and Japan. Over time, various investigations resulted in the retractions of more than 60 studies. However, an analysis by Grey et al.[23] of the approaches used by the four universities, indicated that their investigations were inadequate, difficult to understand, and badly conducted. In a follow-up letter,[24] Grey et al. noted that several of the universities had not addressed the issue of ethical oversight. Indeed, two reported that there were no ethics committees in place at the time of their investigations.

These findings raise an important question: Where is the oversight of research practices? What are the penalties for non-compliance, other than retraction, loss of one's position, and in extreme cases, fines and repayment of grant funds Is anyone ever demoted, say from a full professorship to an associate or assistant? (I have never read of such a penalty, although tenure may prevent it.) In the case of a violation of reporting rules in ClinicalTrials.gov, the Food and Drug Administration Act of 2007 allows fines of up to $10,000 daily for overdue reporting, *but it appears that such fines have never been imposed.*[25]

# Has the FDA Been Helpful in Addressing Misconduct?

What has the FDA been doing? Not much, according to an investigation[26] by the journal Science. The journal's investigators, using the Freedom of Information Act, obtained the results of some 1600 agency inspections and enforcement documents. In one case, a clinician who had obtained contracts focused on pharmacology research, was found to have committed serious lapses in obtaining informed consent, had used unqualified staff to assess medical problems, and had backdated records that were contradictory and disorganized. The FDA asserted that these deviations might constitute both fraud and violations of human subject protections, so warned the investigator that he could be fined and disqualified from conducting trials. Nevertheless, the same problems recurred in multiple subsequent inspections, yet the FDA did not inform the companies sponsoring the trials, did not publicize the findings, and did not tell the subjects their well-being might have been compromised. These lack of FDA sanctions apparently freed the investigator to continue obtaining research contracts with Pharma, which paid his company millions over an 11-year period. He is now recruiting subjects for nine new trials.

The number of FDA-instituted disqualifications of investigators fell from a little more than 10 in President Obama's first 3 years to about half that in his last 3 years, and to two in President Trump's first 3 years. The number of warning letters followed the same pattern, as did cases labeled as "official action indicated." Of 291 instances of the latter, only 71 led to a clear regulatory endpoint. Dozens of these cases took from 10 months to 14 years before a warning letter was issued, probably increasing the risk to subjects. Subjects in several trials were never warned about serious violations of their rights. The *Science* investigation also found that several researchers who had been disqualified by the FDA still took in massive amounts of money from Pharma, ranging from $422,000 to $665,000.

Have the state medical boards taken any action to remedy the problems? After all, medical boards across the United States are obligated to take legal action against their licensees known to have endangered, injured, or behaved inappropriately or illegally toward patients. However, Wolfe et al.,[27] calculated the rate of serious disciplinary actions per 1,000 physicians in each state, gathering data from the National Practitioner Data Bank (NPDB), an organization to which state boards report all such actions. The board actions occurred during the years 2017–2019. Serious actions included suspension of licenses, revocations, summary restrictions, voluntary surrenders of licenses, and refusal of renewals. The average annual rate of serious actions was highest in Kentucky, at 2.29/1000 physicians per year, while the rate in The District of Columbia was last, at 0.29/1000 physicians. The authors concluded that many, or perhaps most, of the stated boards are doing a "dangerously lax job" of enforcing the laws. They also note an unpublished analysis by one of the authors showing that over 8,000 physicians had incurred 5 or more reports of malpractice in 1990–2009, but 76% of these had never suffered a board action of any kind!

In the meantime, scandals continue to emerge, as in the case of the founder of Insys Theraputics, who was convicted of racketeering conspiracy in a federal court in 2019.[28] The founder and four former employees were accused of bribing physicians to boost sales of a fentanyl spray. Their tactic: Paying physicians fees for sham educational sessions, and using a video in which employees, including an exotic dancer, were partying around a huge bottle of fentanyl spray. On a wider front, Perdue Pharma has agreed to plead guilty[29] to criminal charges resulting from its marketing of Oxycontin, and is facing penalties of some $8.3 billion. The owners are looking at $225 million in civil fines, an amount that represents about 2% of the family's net worth. As of December 2020, the family still denies any wrongdoing or responsibility for the opioid epidemic.[30] This has not changed.

Insys Theraputics and Perdue are not the only companies spending huge sums of money on marketing. The U.S. Attorney's Office in the Southern District of New York announced in July of 2020 that Novartis Pharmaceuticals paid $678 million to settle a civil lawsuit that alleged a decade-long pattern of violations of the federal false claims act and the Anti-Kickback Statute.[31] The violations entailed providing physicians with cash payments, recreational outings, and lavish meals in order to increase sales of the company's drugs for diabetes and cardiovascular conditions. In addition, Novartis sponsored thousands of sham educational programs, and paid speakers exorbitant fees for delivering meaningless lectures. In some cases, the company paid doctors for events that never occurred! In addition to the $678 million, Novartis signed a 5-year corporate integrity agreement, agreed to restrict the number of sponsored events, and agreed that the events will take place in virtual formats. The Justice Department stressed that these tactics threatened the impartiality of medical decision making and the financial integrity of Medicare and Medicaid. Note that no executives or employees faced criminal charges, although it was clear that these tactics had been approved by top managers.

# Fraud and Misconduct in Science: Are There Any Realistic Solutions?

I think not. We opened this volume with an account of a number of flagrant instances of misconduct at major academic centers, with all occurring during the past several years, despite the many articles, books, and guidelines aimed at reining in such behavior. What is the central problem? Money. We have a health system that is profit driven from top to bottom, and the financial gains are enormous, not only for the companies, but for stockholders, care-givers, and investigators, all of whom operate in a highly competitive system aimed at maximizing profit and income. Just one segment, the private insurance industry, directly and indirectly employs over 500,000 people, resulting in at least 25% of the health care dollars going to managing the business of medical care. This is a huge source of income for the largest companies, including Aetna, Anthem, Cigna, Humana, and UnitedHealth Group. These five companies saw a quintupling of their stock value between 2010 and 2017.[32, p.125] However, they contribute to the roughly $750 billion lost every year to administrative excess, medical fraud, and lack of significant efforts at prevention.[32, p.4] Spending on personal health care in the United States between 1996 and 2013 increased to at least $1.2 trillion, with spending on depression reaching $71 billion in 2013, $29 billion on anxiety disorders, $23 billion on ADHD, and $17 billion on schizophrenia, for a total of $140 billion on four psychiatric disorders.[33]

Given the money involved, who in the medical-industrial complex wants to change the system to make it more cost-effective and available at lower costs to the public? Instead, the industry is contributing large funds of money aimed maintaining and expanding its grip on the system. Indeed, during the years 1999–2018,[34] Pharma and the health products industries spent $4.9 billion on lobbying at the federal level, an amount greater than expended by any other industry. But this didn't stop at the federal level. The industry also contributed $877 million to state candidates and committees, and $214 million to congressional candidates. (For additional details regarding industry payments to physicians, physician-editors, and medical society leaders, please see Chapter 2.)

In addition, the COVID-19 pandemic has vastly increased the profits of the major health insurers in the second quarter of 2020.[35] UnitedHealth Group in 2019 reported profits of $3.4 billion, increasing to $6.4 billion in 2020, while Anthem reported profits of $1.1 billion in 2019, increasing to $2.3 billion in 2020. Humana had $948 million in profits in 2019, and $1.3 billion in 2020. (Keep in mind these are profits from one quarter!) It appears that the rise in profits was due, at least in part, to the fact that potential patients were skipping their appointments and postponing procedures, either by choice or the mandated shutdown of hospital services due to the demand for COVID beds. The profits are not illegal, but are they appropriate, considering the overall damage to the economy, severe job loss, and millions of people lined up at food banks? And, in July 2020, 20% of physicians had their salaries skipped or deferred, and 24% reported recent layoffs, while many are becoming positive for COVID-19.

Whatever the damage to the population as a whole, the money continues to flow, as found in a brief history of Novavax,[36] which 18 months ago was on the brink of delisting by NASDAQ following the failure of a second failed vaccine trial in less than 3 years. (The company had never brought a vaccine to market.) The stock fell to less than $1/share. However, it was one of seven vaccine makers to win funding from Operation Warp Speed—some $2 billion—which sent its stock up to $80.71 in October 2020. Nevertheless, its efforts to make a vaccine based on harvesting the spike protein from moth cells seemed very promising, as noted in detail by an article in Science.[36] Yet questions arose when the top managers at Novavax made tens of millions from exercising stock options. Two board members pulled in almost $17 million in August 2020, while in September, four senior managers sold $18.9 million in shares. No one has been charged with misconduct.

In another instance, a company attempted to sell 500,000 respirators to the state of Minnesota, with the packaging claiming that the devices were 3M Model 1860.[37] In fact, the devices were not only counterfeit, but the price was far above the usual retail price! The state is investigating, while the company that sold the masks is claiming that an unnamed supplier is at fault, while complying with a cease-and-desist order directing it to reclaim the fake masks.

In another example of pandemic-induced profits,[38] AstraZeneca obtained a $1.2 billion commitment from the government for vaccine development in May, while reporting more than $$3.6 billion in profits from the first half of 2020. Yet the company proceeded to increase prices on a number of its best-selling drugs by some 6%. AstraZeneca was not alone, despite vows from President Trump to curtail the rising cost of medications. Indeed, the 15 largest drug companies in 2020 posted list price increases of 6%–9%,[37] while the rate of inflation was about 1%. It is not clear what the final impact will be, since list prices are subject to negotiation.

# Conclusions

There is no doubt that some sectors of science have made serious attempts to curb the impact of money on research, publication practices, and transparency. We have ClinicalTrials.gov, and the Open Payments database, as well as a growing list of guidelines and standards for journal editors and publishers, including a relatively new field, Journalology. Much more attention is being devoted to peer review, and how to improve it. Yet we have found the rise of predatory journals, an increase in direct-to-consumer advertising, and ongoing industry payments to physicians aimed at selling company products. Some investigators, directly linked to hedge-fund managers, have been passing along early trial results. As described in the introduction, we have seen blatant instances of fraud and misconduct at major academic medical centers,

I have to conclude that our attempts at balancing the risk–benefit ratio and prescribing on a rational basis are being seriously undermined by these behaviors, which are not likely to improve, given the fact that our health care system is driven by profits, from top to bottom. Indeed, money for medical marketing in the United States during the years 1997–2016 had an astounding growth in multiple areas. Here is a summary, as found by Schwartz and Woloshin,[39] with expenditures growing from 1997 to 2016:

- *DTCA*: $2.9 billion to $9.6 billion
- *DTCA prescription drug advertising*: $1.3 billion to $6 billion
- *Money spent on disease awareness campaign*: $177 million to $430 million
- *DTCA for health services by hospitals, dental, mental health centers, cancer centers, home health care, addiction clinics*: $541 million to $2.9 billion
- *Marketing to health care professionals*: $15.6 billion to $20.3 billion, including
  - $5.6 billion for prescriber detailing
  - $13.5 billion for free samples
  - $979 million for direct payments to physicians related to specific drugs
  - $59 million for disease education
- *Number of professional and consumer promotional materials submitted to the FDA for review*: 34, 182 to 97, 252, but the number of violation letters submitted by the FDA fell from 156 to 11!

Although Pharma paid over $11 billion in fines to settle 103 cases involving off-label or deceptive marketing from 1997 on, the FTC took only one action—against a cancer center. Despite the fines, the FDA has continued to advance the wealth of Pharma during the years 1984–2018,[40] by increasing the number of new drug approvals from 34 in 1990–1999 to 41 in 2010–2018. The FDA has also increased the proportion of new drugs approved under the Orphan Drug from 18% in 1984–1995 to 41% in 2008–2018, and has shortened the time for approval of new drugs from 3 years in 1983 to less than 1 year in 2017. The use of Priority Review approvals increased to 81% in 2018. None of this should be surprising, since user fees collected from Pharma increased from an annual mean of $66 million in 1993–1997 to $820 million in 2013–2017. User fees have been shown to account for some 80% of the salaries paid to staffers who approve new drug applications.[37] On the face of it, this seems a remarkable conflict of interest.

But kudos to the FDA[41] for sending warning letters to Pfizer, Eli Lilly, and others regarding their increasing use of social media to market their drugs, Forest Laboratories, for example, has provided links to donepezil, escitalopram, and memantine, but, like many similar cases, failed to provide generic names of the drugs, information on adverse events, and poor information regarding indications. Other companies are using video postings on Facebook and MySpace for DTCA. Note, however, that the cited article was published in 2009, so it seems doubtful that the letters had any substantial effect.

I submit that scientific misconduct and fraud cannot be significantly remedied in the absence of a nation-wide, single-payer health plan. Yet, I have to admit that similar problems have just been revealed in Great Britain—despite the National Health Service—where some 1,200 government contracts worth almost $22 billion aimed at fighting COVID-19 were rushed out, hoping to rapidly obtain personal protective equipment and other supplies. However, an investigation by the *New York Times*[42] found that about $11 billion went to companies headed by friends of the Conservative Party, or companies with no prior experience, but were closely tied politically. Almost half of the contracts dealt in the first 7 months remain hidden from the public.

However, the United States is not free of similar problems, as noted by a 2021 report by McCoy et al.[43] McCoy's team investigated 11 years of personal financial disclosures by all members of Congress, then calculated the percentage of members holding a health-related asset. The median total value per member was $43,000, but, surprisingly, the assets of members of health care-focused committees and subcommittees did not differ from other members. The total value of these assets ranged from $34 million in 2004–2005 to $64 million in 2013. However, these assets totaled less than 4% of the member's overall financial holding. (Note that limitations on disclosure prevented gathering of data beyond 2014.) The authors recommended that much more attention be paid to COIs in Congress, given the its power to set health-related policies. Unfortunately, the authors could not assess possible correlations between health care assets and legislative activity.

Once again, money and power rule, so misconduct and fraud will continue Making matters worse, we now have evidence that the brain adapts to dishonesty. A study in *Nature Neuroscience*,[44] using fMRI, found a reduction in signaling from the amygdala in the context of dishonesty, The degree of reduced sensitivity to dishonesty then predicted an escalation of self-serving dishonesty in the next decision! This seems to support the idea of a slippery slope, wherein relatively small episodes of misconduct an escalate into larger and more serious episodes. If this finding is replicated, it adds urgency to the need for prevention of and a faster response to misconduct, instead of waiting for more egregious cases.

In the next and final chapter, we will shine more light on the transition to a business-oriented, entrepreneurial medical system that is even more closely aligned with industry. What does this portend for patients, clinicians, and rational prescribing?

# References

1. Broad, W, Wade, N. *Betrayers of the Truth: Fraud and Deceit in the Halls of Science*. Simon & Shuster, New York, 1982.
2. Goodstein, D. Scientific fraud. *American Scholar*, Autumn 1991, pp. 505–515.
3. Judson, HF. *The Great Betrayal. Fraud in Science*. Harcourt, Inc., Orlando, 2004.
4. Gross, C Scientific misconduct. *Annual Review of Psychology* 2016. https://doi.org/10.1146/annurev-psych-122114-033437
5. National Science Foundation. 1996. *Research Misconduct*. National Science Foundation, Arlington, VA. https://www.nsf.gov/oig/resmisreg.pdf (Accessed November 13, 2020).

6. Swazey, JP, et al. Ethical problems in academic research. *American Science* 1993.
7. Kalichman, MW, et al. A pilot study of biomedical trainees' perceptions concerning research ethics. *Academic Medicine* 1992.
8. Titus, SL, et al. Repairing research integrity. *Nature* 2008.
9. Fanelli, D. How many scientists fabricate and falsify research? A systematic review and meta-analysis of survey data. *Public Library of Science One* 2009.
10. Geggie, DA. Survey of newly appointed consultants' attitudes toward research fraud. *Journal of Medical Ethics* 2001.
11. Rahman, H, et al. Dishonesty and research misconduct within the medical profession. *BioMed Central Medical Ethics* 2020. https://doi.org/101186/s12910-020-0461-z
12. Artino, AR Jr, et al. Ethical shades of gray: international frequency of scientific misconduct and questionable research practices in health professions education. *Academic Medicine* 2019.
13. Steen, RG. Retractions in the scientific literature: is the incidence of research fraud increasing. *Journal of Medical Ethics* 2011.
14. Resnik, DV, et al. Scientific retractions and corrections related to misconduct findings. *Journal of Medical Ethics* 2013.
15. Shuchtman, M. Stopping the slide to research fraud. *Canadian Medical Association Journal* 2017. https://doi.org/10.1053/cmaj.1095387
16. Conroy, G. Is research integrity training a waste of time? *Nature Index* 2020. Available at: natureindex.com/news/blog/is-research-integrity-a-waste-of-time
17. Marusic, A, et al. Interventions to prevent misconduct and promote integrity in research and publication. *Cochrane Database of Systematic Reviews* 2016. https://doi.org/10.1002/14651858.MR000038.pub2
18. Kornfield, DS. Perspective: research misconduct: the search for a remedy. *Academic Medicine* 2012.
19. Phillips, T, et al. America COMPETES at 5 years: an analysis of research-intensive universities' RCT training plans. *Science and Engineering Ethics* 2018.
20. Satalkar, P, et al. How do researchers acquire and develop notions of research integrity? A qualitative study among biomedical researchers in Switzerland. *BioMed Central Medical Ethics* 2019. https://doi.org/10.1186/s12910-019-0410-x
21. Nature Index. British universities fail at research integrity self-regulation. https://www.natureindex.com/news-blog/british-universities-fail-at-research-integrity-self-regulation
22. Else, H. What universities can learn from an epic case of research fraud. Analysis of misconduct suggests institutional probes aren't rigorous enough. *Nature* 2019.
23. Grey, A, et al. Quality of reports of investigations of research integrity by academic institutions. *Research Integrity and Peer Review* 2019.
24. Grey, A, et al. Evaluating ethics oversight during assessment of research integrity. *Research Integrity and Peer Review* 2019. https://doi.org/10.1186/s41073-019-0028-6
25. Anderson, ML, et al. Compliance with results reporting at ClinicalTrials.Gov. *New England Journal of Medicine* 2015.
26. Piller, C. Official inaction. A science investigation shows that the FDA oversight of clinical trials is lax, slow-moving, and secretive—and that enforcement is declining. *Science* 2020.
27. Wolfe, S, et al. Ranking of the rate of state medical board's serious disciplinary actions, 2017–2019. *Public Citizen*, March 31, 2007.
28. Richer, AD. Ex-CEO guilty in opioid bribery case. *Minneapolis Star Tribune* 2019.
29. Hoffman, J, et al. Purdue admits that it pushed deadly opioid. A guilty plea and an $8 billion settlement. *New York Times*, October 22, 2020.
30. Hoffman, J. Grilled by Congress, sacklers deny responsibility for opioid epidemic. *New York Times*, 2020.
31. Press release. The United States Attorney's Office, Southern District of New York. *Acting Manhattan U.S, Attorney announces $678 million settlement of fraud lawsuit against Novartis Pharmaceutical Corporation.* Wednesday, July 1, 2020.

32. MaGee, M. *Code Blue. Inside America's Medical Industrial Complex.* Atlantic Monthly Press, New York, 2019.
33. Dieleman, JL, et al. U.S. spending on personal health care and public health. *JAMA* 2016.
34. Wouters, OJ. Lobbying expenditures and campaign contributions by the pharmaceutical and health product industry in the United States, 1998–2018. *JAMA Internal Medicine* 2020. https://doi.org/10.1001/jamainternmed.2020.0416
35. Holpuch, A. US health insurers double profits in second quarter amid pandemic. *Guardian*, US Edition, August 14, 2020.
36. Wadman, M. The long shot. A little company chases its biggest competitors in the race for a corona virus vaccine. *Science* 2020.
37. Carlson, J. Firm surrenders 500K fake masks. *Minneapolis Star Tribune*, December 23, 2020.
38. Leveys, N. Despite aid from feds, AstraZeneca hikes prices. The company has said it would not profit from pandemic vaccine sales. *Minneapolis Star Tribune*, Business Section, September 16, 2020. (Reprinted from the *Los Angeles Times*.)
39. Schwartz, LM, et al. Medical marketing in the United States, 1996–2016. *JAMA* 2019. https://doi.org/10.1001/jama.2018.19320
40. Darrow, JJ, et al. FDA approval and regulation of pharmaceuticals, 1983–2018. *JAMA* 2020. https://doi.org/10.1001/jama.2019.20288
41. Yan, J FDA catching up with drug companies that push online envelope. *Psychiatric News* 2009. https://doi.org/10.1176/pn.44.11.0004a
42. Bradley, J, et al. Waste, negligence and cronyism in Britain's pandemic response. *New York Times*, December 18, 2020.
43. McCoy, M, et al. Historical trends in health care-related financial holdings among members of Congress. *Public Library of Science One* 2021. https://doi.org/10.1371/journal.pone.0253624
44. Garrett, N, et al. The brain adapts to dishonesty. *Nature Neuroscience* 2016. https://doi.org/10.1038/nn.4426

# 11

# An Entrepreneurial Health Care System
## Risks and Benefits to Rational Prescribing

## Introduction

In the preceding 10 chapters, our focus has been on the many steps taken by Pharma to influence the academic agenda, steps that have largely been successful due to the remarkable growth in wealth of the industry. As we have noted, this has led to generous research and non-research payments to individual clinicians, editors of scientific journals, medical societies, and editorial boards, all in an attempt to influence the research agenda, study outcomes, and a remarkable increase in profits over the decades. Unfortunately, these efforts have also led to an escalation of drug costs, and a health care system that is the most costly in the world, but ranks among the worst when it comes to access to care, administrative efficiency, and health care outcomes.[1-3] We have documented as well a steady stream of misconduct and outright fraud in some of our most prestigious institutions, as well as a host of other behaviors that undermine the ability of clinicians to appropriately address the risk–benefit ratio of their treatments. These include suppression of negative studies, spin, changing or omitting primary outcomes, and fraudulent authorship. Yet in some instances the Food and Drug Administration (FDA) has failed to take corrective actions, nor have state licensing boards. Nevertheless, we are now witnessing a move to foster ever closer ties between academia and industry, accompanied by the development of new operational and financial models that could benefit both sectors.[4] As Alice Lam put it in 2010,[5] this involves a transition from "ivory tower traditionalists," who embrace strict boundaries between academia and industry, to a field perhaps dominated by "entrepreneurial scientists." Her paper contains more than 60 citations, none of which include the many journals cited in this volume, such as *JAMA*, *Lancet*, or any psychiatry or psychology journals, perhaps indicative of the split that she explores and encourages.

## Roots of Change

We have documented the foundations of this change in the rise of academic capitalism in the Introduction and Chapter 1 of this volume (see for citations), with the development and marketing of antipsychotics, antidepressants, and antianxiety agents playing a major role. We also noted the regulatory and legislative initiatives such as the Bayh-Dole Act in 1980, an act that clearly fostered the growth of ties between academia and industry, as did the Hatch-Waxman Act that added years of patent protection. The 1951 decree by the FDA that required

DOI: 10.1201/9781003267218-12

prescriptions for new medications, also gave Pharma an opportunity to expand its research agenda, as did the dramatic expansion of psychiatric diagnoses in 1980. In 1997, the FDA loosened its restrictions on direct-to-consumer advertising. By 2002, the profit margins of the top ten pharmaceutical companies exceeded those of any other industry.

The rise of advocacy groups such as the National Alliance for the Mentally Ill (NAMI) afforded Pharma another opportunity to expand its clout by providing financial support for such groups. For example, the Heart Rhythm Society in 2010 collected some $16 million,[6] almost half of which came from drug and device makers, although the Society denied that the money had any influence on its policies. However, 12 of its 18 board members were paid speakers or consultants to the companies, an arrangement similar to that found in the American Society of Hypertension, where 12 of 14 board members had financial ties to industry. In addition, Daiichi Sankyo, the ASH's largest donor, gave the organization over $3.3 million in 2009, no doubt a good investment since the company makes a number of anti-hypertensive agents. The ASH also ran a training program for Daiichi sales representatives,[6] allowing them to print cards noting that they are ASH accredited!

More ties include those between the National Lipid Association (NLA), and six companies that could profit from the NLA's recommendations on screening and treatment.[7] In the United Kingdom, the Royal Institute of Blind People recommended against the use of a less expensive medication (Avastin) for the treatment of macular degeneration, although Lucentis at that time was 40 times as expensive. Interestingly, Novartis, the maker of Lucentis and Avastin, was a supporter of the Royal Institute, but the Institute claimed that the contributions from Novartis amounted to only 1% of all donations.[7]

These probable COIs were cited in articles published in 2011, but many of the studies we cited in Chapter 2 were published in 2018–2020, indicating that the early warnings and concerns had gone unappreciated. For example, another analysis of doctor's ties to Pharma and the impact on Medicare prescribing was published in 2019,[8] with results similar to those of Sharma et al. in 2018.[9] In the 2019 study by Fresques et al.,[8] physicians who had interactions, usually in the form of general payments (non-research) from the manufacturers of the 50 most-prescribed brand-name drugs in Medicare Part D, prescribed these drugs at higher rates than physicians who had no such interactions. Note that 38 of the 50 drugs had yearly costs to the patient exceeding $1,000, although that may have changed over time. Unfortunately, one in five doctors who prescribed Oxycontin under Medicare had a promotional interaction with Purdue Pharma.[8]

## COIs in guideline authors

As the interest in evidence-based medicine grew, so did the development of clinical practice guidelines, but multiple studies have shown that financial COIs (FCOIs) between guideline authors and industry have long been known to result in higher rates of prescriptions for expensive brand name drugs and more recommendations for drugs manufactured by the company.[10] Let's examine a few guidelines, their authors, and their financial entanglements. Payments to guideline authors are present across cancer,[10] otolaryngology,[11] and gastroenterology,[12] to name a few. Regarding specific payments, there is considerable variation, but some are quite large:

- *Cancer guidelines:*[10] Eighty-six percent of 125 guideline authors had at least one FCOI. They received an average of $10,011 in general payments for meals, lodging, and $236, 006 in research payments. Six percent had FCOIs in excess of $50,000 net.
- *Otolaryngology guidelines:*[11] Of 49 authors, 80% received an industry payment. 43% accepted more than $1000; 24% more than $50,000, and 4% more than $100,000.

The mean payment was $18, 431 per physician. Disclosure statements disagreed with data from Open Payments in three cases.

- *Gastroenterology guidelines:*[12] Twenty-nine of 36 clinical guidelines included panelists who accepted honoraria or consultation fees from industry. Of these, 22% accepted payments of $10,000 or more.

If we look at individual payments to 15,497 gastroenterologists,[12] we find that 86.9% of received more than 422,000 payments totaling $67144,862. Similarly, in 2007,[13] orthopedic device makers made 1,041 payments totaling $198 million to 939 orthopedic surgeons. After a landmark settlement with the Department of Justice in 2008, the device makers made 568 payments to orthopedic surgeons, but increased the total to $228 million! The proportion of orthopedic surgeons with academic affiliations who received payments rose from 39.4% in 2007 to 44.9% in 2008.

Despite these obvious FCOIs and their impact on prescribing and costs, Lam in 2010[5] emphasized that scientists themselves have been actively engaged in shaping the relationship between science and businesses, while universities have become willing actors in the move to exploit academic research in order to become competitors in the knowledge market and enhance their revenue. In Minneapolis, for example, the chair of the University of Minnesota gave a Grand Rounds at the Minneapolis VA Medical Center in the mid-1990s, and described in detail the numbers of faculty with grants from various institutions and companies. One VA investigator then stood up and asked: What were the goals and results? The answers were vague. Unfortunately, his message was not unique, as Campbell et al.[14] demonstrated in a survey of 688 department chairs, of whom 459 responded. Sixty percent acknowledged a personal relationship with industry, serving as a paid speaker, consultant, founder, or member of a board of directors.

Fast forward to September 18, 2021, when the President of the University of Minnesota, Joan Gable, and two regents published an op-ed [15] in which they boasted of an all-time high in new startup companies and record-breaking funding of more than $1 billion, including record-breaking philanthropic support. However, they did note "ground-breaking" work in agriculture, early childhood development, and solutions aimed at solving problems in transportation, Remarkably, for a state with a strong indigenous population, the University had the "first-ever" meeting with the Minnesota Indian Affairs Council. What were the results? What portion of the $1 billion came from the drug industry? Were there COIs in the grant recipients?

However, despite the enthusiasm, some investigators have opposed this transition, and have warned of the institutional risks associated with academic entrepreneurialism, as we have shown in Chapters 1 and 10. In addition, an editorial in 2004[16] cited the widespread criticism of the academic-industrial relationship, as did Moncrief in 2007,[17] and Becker,[18] who noted in 2020 a study[19] showing that 18 health care leaders who had served on an industry board for a full year in 2017 received an average compensation package of $475,000, and held company stock worth on average $1.7 million! Well, who would want to reject that kind of prestige and wealth? Not many. Indeed, 17 years prior to the Becker study, Bekelman et al.[20] published a systematic review of FCOIs in biomedical research, and found that about 25% of investigators had affiliations with industry, and two-thirds of academic institutions held equity in start-ups performed at those institutions, while industry sponsorship tripled pro-industry conclusions. In addition, such sponsorship was associated with restrictions on data-sharing and publication, a problem noted as well by Blumenthal et al.,[21] who found that 19.8% of academic life scientists reported a delay in publication of more than 6 months at least once in the past 3 years. The delay was needed to allow time for patent application, or to resolve disputes over ownership of intellectual property. Almost 9% reported refusing to share research results with other scientists.

## Collaboration between universities and industry

In 2014, Julia Haller[22] noted that academic ties to industry are not new, and in fact date to the 1920s and 1930s when the Massachusetts Institute of Technology (MIT) began to interact with non-academic entities that focused on chemical engineering and the developed of new models of patenting and licensing relevant to their discoveries. MIT went on to collaborate with Standard Oil, while similar relationships began at the Universities of Wisconsin and Illinois. MIT consultants rotated in and out of Standard Oil, whose refinery served as a laboratory for MIT students. MIT also began an agreement with the Research Corporation in 1937 that expanded its patent and licensing activities, although the benefits were less than expected. Nevertheless, the Bayh-Dole Act, as we have stressed several times, pushed such collaborations forward. For example, Novartis developed an exclusionary relationship with the University of California at Berkeley, while UC San Francisco developed partnerships with Sanofi and Pfizer, and GlaxoSmithKline began putting academic scientists from the University of Cambridge into their laboratories.

While Haller notes[22] that perhaps half of these early collaborative projects yielded major outcomes, the "benefits are incontrovertible." Indeed, Freedman and Mullane in 2017 documented a host of similar interactions,[4] first stating that medical research has "dumped any pretense of social altruism," and has embraced big business! The authors went on to trace the steps of this transition, many of which we have already described. However, they note that discoveries by academic scientists had long been plagued by the lack of skill and resources in marketing discoveries, thus adding to the push for collaboration. Indeed, academic translational centers have blossomed, including the Clinical and Translational Science Institute at the University of California San Francisco, the Institute for Translational Medicine and Therapeutics at the University of Pennsylvania, as well as several others. On the business side, we have seen the appearance of Small Business Innovation Research and Small Business Technology Transfer awards, while The Rockefeller Institute created the Robertson Therapeutic Development Fund with a $25 million dollar gift from the Robertson Foundation.[4]

Academic drug discovery centers are also emerging. Note the appearance in 2013 of the Academic Drug Discovery Consortium that by 2016 had 141 affiliated centers, including the Conrad Prebys Center for Chemical Genomics at the Sanford Burnham Prebys Center for Chemical Genomics, and the California Institute for Biomedical Research.[4] Companies have also allied themselves with a specific research institute, with Eli Lilly, Johnson & Johnson, Novartis, and Pfizer establishing partnerships with the Scripps Research Institute. Note that Scripps entered into a 10-year agreement on 1997 with Novartis in return for $200 million, and a 5-year agreement with Pfizer for $100 million in 2006. Similar agreements were signed between Monsanto, the University of Washington, and the Harvard Medical School.

The authors also take note of open innovation (OI) as a new model[4] in which specific needs or problems are put out to the community, often on a competitive basis. Help is also sought from crowd-sourcing, a model that began with the Eli Lilly development of InnoCentive, a web-based platform aimed at gathering input from a global network of problem solvers. This was followed by similar efforts from Pfizer and other companies, foundations, and government agencies. Sage Bionetworks has used this model to develop complex predictive models of disease, while others have used it to investigate structures of proteins.

In 2021, Costa et al.[23] stressed that academics in recent years have developed a keen interest in open innovation, viewing it as a catalyst of knowledge production, diffusion of information, while stimulating greater collaboration with industry. Companies implement OI via multiple sources, including universities, suppliers, research institutes, and even competitors, resulting in an "unbounded" OI strategy critical to the entrepreneurial vision the universities and companies. The common link between industry and the university is technology transfer, with universities serving as important sources of scientific information.

## Academic Centers and Economic Advantages from Collaboration?

But what is the economic advantage? Does OI result in improved financial performance? If so, to whom? The authors[23] developed an extensive database of companies, their performance, and whether they were involved in collaboration with universities. An econometric analysis found that connecting to a university raised financial performance by 57.7%, with another 36% gain from each university contacted, which seems overblown, since the company could see gains of over 100% if connected with three. In general, OI and university-industry-collaboration (UIC) are mutually reinforcing, but note that in this lengthy and complex analysis, the focus is on the financial advantages to companies. Indeed, the authors stress that governments should encourage academic innovation as a foundation for economic development. The university system "must" contribute to society through the creation, transfer of knowledge, and technologies, which necessitates a change from the traditional university structure to a corporate structure.[23] The authors appear to assume that the growth in industrial financial performance will trickle down to the university and then to the public, and perhaps to the individual, although the public and the clinician are not mentioned. Nevertheless, we have established that industry payments to individual physicians, editors, board members and others have been impressively high in some instances, but what of the academic medical center itself?

In 2017, three deans of research-intensive universities published an editorial[24] in which they observe that the lack of financial support for education and a fall-off in research support from the NIH have understandably led institutional leaders to seek funding from industry, endowments, and the like, leading academic centers to become increasingly businesslike. This has taken the form of mergers, purchase of community hospitals, and the establishment of health-care networks. Similarly, drug companies and device makers have indulged in mergers and acquisitions, yet some have downsized their research and development programs, but at the same hope to discover potential blockbusters such as fluoxetine (Prozac).

Yet the authors stress that the move to commercialize discoveries via the collaboration of academic medical centers and industry has not resulted in significant gains in wealth. Indeed, only 2% of patents yield as much as $1 million per year, and even fewer accrue $100 million. Nevertheless, the authors insist that such relationships can be mutually beneficial, if academic leaders manage COIs, and avoid putting excessive pressure on the faculty to seek patents or emphasize discoveries that will succeed in the marketplace.[24]

Is this practical, given the competition for grants, promotions, and prestige? Indeed, a lengthy essay in the journal Science,[25] published in September 2021, noted that the processes by which academic promotions and tenure (P&T) are determined may fail to fully assess and value the innovative/entrepreneurial work now in high demand at universities. In an effort to correct this oversight, we now have a Promotion and Tenure-Innovation and Entrepreneurialship Coalition (PTIE) comprised of over 65 universities and many stakeholder organizations, including the National Science Foundation, which supports the PTIE. The aim of the PTIE is to support a more innovative and diverse professoriate from the fields of science, technology mathematics, and medicine, as well as the liberal arts. These changes may take 5–10 years, as they expand the campus culture. Yet they should not undermine, supplant, or dilute basic and/or curiosity-driven research, a primary mission of the university. Nevertheless, in this new and expanded university culture, the focus appears to be on research that has an impact on the social contract. Given that aim, it's difficult to see how basic and curiosity-driven research can compete for funding and prestige.

Others have proposed steps that could make these goals possible, with Moses et al.[26] 20 years ago recommending four principles:

- Veracity of research results, whether clinical or basic, cannot be compromised.
- A disinterested party should provide oversight.
- Control of intellectual property and proprietary rights should be openly acknowledged at the outset, with minimal restrictions on nondisclosure.
- Financial and nonfinancial incentives should address he needs of the institution, senior investigators and the junior faculty.

How to accomplish these goals? By way of a separate research institute, additional external oversight, and/or the creation of a new entity separate from the university to receive royalties and hold equity. None of these can be found in the PTIE paper.

# Conclusions

While numerous authors have made suggestions that might lessen the negative impact of collaboration with industry, the studies we have cited throughout this volume suggest that the drive for funding and prestige has not only continued but worsened, with a substantial impact on drug prices and COIs. We have noted repeatedly studies that demonstrate better outcomes secondary to industry sponsorship and collaboration with university investigators. How can this be otherwise, since the pharmaceutical industry and device makers have the money, and their primary responsibility is to their boards and shareholders, not to their collaborators in academic medical centers. While open innovation has its attractive features, it also invites even more entities into the collaborative field of play, perhaps further diluting the academic power structure—despite assurances from OI enthusiasts.

In many of the recent papers on these developments, little is said about the effects of the entrepreneurial surge on clinicians and patients. The evidence at this point shows that collaboration with industry skews outcomes in favor of industry, and thus skews the risk–benefit ratio, making rational prescribing more difficult. I find it remarkable that even following the establishment of the Open Payments database, and years of criticism regarding pharma's payments to physicians, the industry in 2015 sent $235 million in food and beverage payments to physicians, although the mean value was per physician was only $400.[27] On the other hand, it has been well established that even a single meal can increase the prescribing rate of a branded drug.[28]

Will increasing the depth and breadth of the academic industry collaboration serve to correct such behaviors? I doubt it. It seems far more likely that COIs will become more widespread, given the added complexities of the entrepreneurial paradigm, and the number of entities involved, thus making rational prescribing even more difficult, and increasing health care costs.

# References

1. McGee, M. Code blue. Inside America's Medical Industrial Complex. *Atlantic Monthly Press* 2019.
2. Schneider, EC, et al. Mirror, mirror 2021. Reflecting poorly: health care in the U.S. compared to other high-income countries. *Commonwealth Fund*, August 2021.
3. GBD 2016 healthcare access and quality collaborators. *Lancet* 2018. http://dx.doi.org/10.1016/S0140-6736(18)30994-2
4. Freedman, S, et al. The academic-industrial complex: navigating the translational and cultural divide. *Drug Discovery* 2017. http://dx.doi.org/10.1010/j.drudis.2017.03.005
5. Lam, A. From 'Ivory tower traditionalists' to 'entrepreneurial scientists'? *Social Studies of Science* 2010. http://dx.doi.org/10.1177/0306312709349963
6. Ornstein, C, et al. Financial ties bind medical societies to drug and device makers. *ProPublica*, May 5, 2011.
7. Kusnetz, N. Report details more drug industry ties to medical societies. *ProPublica*, May 20, 2011.
8. Fresques, H, et al. How we analyzed doctors' pharma industry ties and Medicare prescribing. *ProPublica*, December 20, 2019.
9. Sharma, M, et al. Association between industry payments and prescribing costly medication: an observational study using open payments and Medicare Part D data. *BioMed Central Health Services Research* 2018. https://doi.org/10.1186/s12913-018-3043-8
10. Mitchell, AP, et al. Financial relationships with industry among national comprehensive cancer network guideline authors. *JAMA Oncology* 2016.
11. Horn, J, et al. Evaluation of industry relationships among authors of otolaryngology clinical practice guidelines. *JAMA Otolaryngology Head Neck Surgery* 2018. https://doi.org/10.1001/jamaoto.2017.2741
12. Nusrat, S, et al. Assessment of pharmaceutical company and device manufacturer payments to gastroenterologists and their participation in clinical practice guideline panels. *JAMA Network Open* 2018. https://doi.org/10.1001/jamanetworkopen.2018.6343
13. Hockenberry, JM, et al. Financial payments by orthopedic device makers to orthopedic surgeons. *Archives of Internal Medicine* 2011.
14. Campbell, EG, et al. Institutional academic-industry relationships. *JAMA* 2007.
15. Gabel, J, et al. U's commitment to state's service has never been stronger. *Minneapolis Star Tribune*, September 18, 2021, p.A7.
16. Norris, J. Industry and academic medicine. *Canadian Journal of Neurology* 2004.
17. Moncrieff, J. Co-opting psychiatry: the alliance between academic psychiatry and the pharmaceutical industry. *Epidemiologica Psihiatria Sociale* 2007. https://doi.10.1017/S112189X00002268
18. Becker, C. Relationships between academic medicine leaders and industry—time for another look? *JAMA* 2020.
19. Dunn, A. Memorial Sloan Kettering scandal raises questions for pharma's biggest corporate boards. *Biopharma Dive* 2018. https://www.biopharmadive.com/news/memorial-sloan-kettering-scandal-raises-questions-for-pharmas-biggest-corp/540750/
20. Bekelman, JE, et al. Scope and impact of financial conflicts of interest in biomedical research. A systematic review. *JAMA* 2003.
21. Blumenthal, D, et al. Withholding research results in academic life science. Evidence from a national survey of faculty. *JAMA* 1997.
22. Haller, JA. Strengthened ties between industry and academia are historical, productive, and crucial. *Survey of Opthalmology* 2014.

23. Costa, J, et al. Two sides of the same coin: university-industry collaboration and open innovation as enhancers of industry performance. *Sustainability* 2021. https://doi.org/10.3390/su13073866

24. Pizzo, PA, et al. Role of leaders in fostering meaningful collaborations between academic medical centers and industry while also managing individual and institutional conflicts of interest. *JAMA* 2017.

25. Carter, R, et al. Innovation, entrepreneurship, promotion, and tenure. Academic incentives must reward broader societal impacts. *Science* 2021.

26. Moses, H, et al. Academic relationships with industry. A new model for biomedical research. *JAMA* 2001.

27. Steinbrook, R. Physicians, industry payments for food and beverages, and drug prescribing. *JAMA* 2017.

28. Dejong, C, et al. Pharmaceutical industry-sponsored meals and physician prescribing patterns for Medicare beneficiaries. *JAMA Internal Medicine* 2016.

# Index